# Skin Diseases of Dogs and Cats

## A Guide for Pet Owners and Professionals

*Dr. Steven A. Melman*

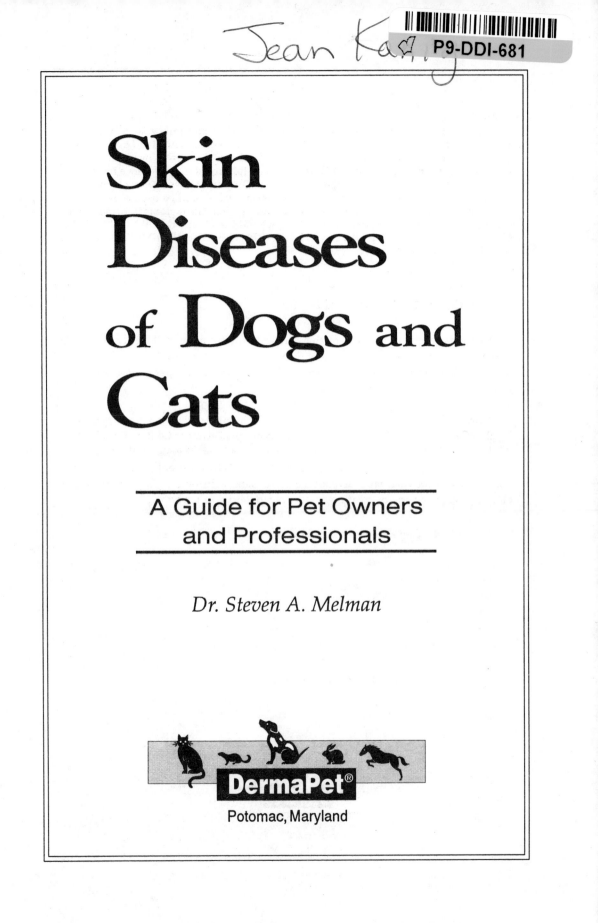

**DermaPet®**

Potomac, Maryland

Notice

Maximum efforts have been expended by the author and publisher to insure the accuracy of dosage recommendations, which are in agreement with standards accepted at the time of publication. Dosage schedules may be changed as new clinical data or more experience with the drug suggest a better protocol. It is urged that reference be made to the manufacturer's recommendations for dosages. Drugs that have been recommended, but are not officially approved for use in a given species should be used only with the knowledge of potential side-effects and with caution after the owner is informed of the experimental nature of the drug. SINCE THIS BOOK IS INTENDED FOR NON-VETERINARIANS, ALWAYS CONSULT A VETERINARIAN BEFORE ATTEMPTING TO USE ANY DRUG OR TREAT ANY DISEASE.

DermaPet®, Inc.
P.O. Box 59713
Potomac, Maryland 20859
Tel. # 301-983-8387

ISBN 0-9640295-0-2

Library of Congress Catalog Card Number: 94-94063

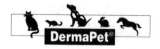

# Dedication

I want to dedicate this book to three special friends: Kingbud, my loyal companion who is mainly a German shepherd; Abigail my basset hound — the sweetest dog to whom anyone ever belonged; and Dinky, my Lhasa apso who is also a sturdy and steadfast companion.

Special thanks for their patience and support to my wife, Gloria, who has tolerated me through it all; and to my truly beautiful daughters, Jessica, who is rapidly becoming quite a writer in her own right, and Stacey, whose persistence will lead her way on the road to success. And lest I forget, I owe quite a lot to DermaPet Inc., which has provided me with the forum, funds and power to publish and distribute this book.

# Contents

# Preface

Ask any practicing veterinarian to name the most common reasons why people bring their pets to the clinic, and most will place skin problems at or near the top of the list. That's not at all surprising when you consider how many very different skin diseases there are, and how incredibly varied the causes of these ailments can be. On top of this, there is a tremendous distress on the part of pet owners who can no longer bear to watch their beloved dogs and cats itch, scratch, lick or chew themselves into miserable shadows of their former selves. And then there is the frustration shouldered by the veterinarian who oftentimes has to put the pet through a detailed work-up and perhaps a variety of trials, tests and therapies before making a final diagnosis. And all the while, the pet owner is asking, "Can't you do something, right now?"

If you have experienced the frustration and sense of helplessness that comes with watching a pet suffer through the discomforts of a skin disease, then you will know how necessary and important a book such as this is. You, more than anybody else, will understand the need for a book that finally explains — in plain English — the whole gamut of skin diseases that can afflict cats and dogs. This book is written specifically for pet owners and professionals who want to know exactly what is afflicting their pets, what's behind the disease, what does the veterinarian have to do to identify both the ailment and its causes, and what can be done to bring about a cure.

But be aware: This work is not expected to be a replacement for professional veterinary care. Rather, it was written to aid the veterinary professional by helping pet owners and professionals reach a greater understanding and appreciation of the tremendous challenges that lie ahead on the road to recovery. This book should help veterinarians explain exactly why various tests are being done, or why healing cannot be expected overnight. When the medical professional and the pet owner share a full awareness of the problems that need to be overcome, they can better cooperate to bring about a healing for the suffering animal.

This book should also prove invaluable to veterinarians who may not have received specific postdoctoral training in the field of veterinary dermatology, and who can therefore appreciate a guide to explain to their clients the direction in which further research is going. It may also be useful in the hands of non-veterinary professionals — such as groomers, veterinary technicians and staff, trainers, kennel operators, breeders, pet store owners and "serious" pet owners — who may wish to "field questions" from worried animal owners before guiding them to seek professional veterinary help. These non-medical professionals can also use this book to learn about and avoid some of the more typical causes of feline and canine dermatological problems.

I cannot overemphasize that *this book is NOT intended as a substitute for a visit to the veterinarian*. Just because various chapters make mention of various medications, most references omit specific protocols regarding dosages, drug interactions, frequency of use and duration of treatment. And as most of our contributing experts point out, many diseases look alike and therefore require consultation from a trained clinician. What this book will do is *help you understand what that clinician is talking about!*

The book begins with chapters on Anatomy and Physiology/Structure and Function, Diagnostic Procedures, Pharmacology and Shampoo Therapy. These are the most important chapters for non-veterinary professionals, since they are the building blocks upon which the remainder of the book stands. A firm understanding of these basics is helpful in better understanding the explanations and procedures outlined throughout the book. This is not to say that you cannot read a section on a specific diagnosis first, and then refer to other sections for a better understanding. Readers will find cross-references throughout the book, and a Glossary of Terms which was compiled from definitions offered by each contributing veterinary expert.

## How This Book Can Help...

### Groomers, Kennel Operators and Pet Retailers

You are on the front line in the battle to keep the nation's pets healthy. Pet owners come to you first, expecting you to help meet their companion animals' hygienic needs, for shelter when necessary, for counsel when training and behavioral problems arise, and for guidance on which products will provide the optimum health. Your role is very important, but you must always be careful about crossing the line and offering advice that is better left to the veterinary professional. You don't want to be diagnosing, treating diseases, or questioning a veterinarian's advice. You may sympathize with a customer whose pet appears to be making little improvement under professional care, but it would not be a very good idea for you to recommend another veterinarian or to overrule the veterinary professional and advise your own treatment program.

Perhaps the best thing you can do is advise the pet owner to see a specialist — one who has special training and experience in the field of veterinary dermatology. This advice may actually help avoid an expensive visit, in some cases. The customer has the right to hear your advice, and you owe it to your customers to recommend they take their pets to a specialist. Of course, nothing stops you from recommending a product you really believe in, such as an ear cleaner. You will know from the chapter on Ear Diseases that cleaning ears can often help avoid future problems, and that the product you are endorsing meets the requirements for doing the job safely and effectively. Just be sure that while you are recommending a product, you are reminding customers that you are not a veterinarian and that you are therefore unable to say for sure what disease is ailing their pets. If your advice helps the pet, and saves the owner a bundle in veterinary bills, you will have won another loyal customer.

### Veterinarians

As a general practitioner, one of the greatest challenges is answering the question: When to refer? That's especially true when it comes to skin diseases, since dermatological ailments make up a majority of cases seen in practice. It can't be denied that too many referrals could lead to serious financial loss. It is also unfortunate that some equate referral with failure. Nothing can be further from the truth. Referral is simply another tool that veterinarians can and should make use of. And that's where this book can be useful, since it will help your clientele understand exactly what challenges you are facing in making a proper diagnosis and prescribing the appropriate treatment. You want your customers to know exactly how difficult skin diseases can be, because in the end it will be their choice as to whether or not they should take the dog to a specialist. It will be your responsibility to say, from the very start, that there are those who have extensive dermatological training and that at some point the pet owner may want to see one. Once your clients understand exactly what they — and you — are up against, they will not be disappointed by your recommendation that they take their dog or cat to a relatively more expensive specialist. Being up front and honest about the possibility of a future referral will help guarantee the customer doesn't ask the specialist: "Why wasn't I sent to you sooner?"

### Veterinary technicians and clinic employees

A veterinary clinic is only successful through the combined efforts of everybody involved, including the veterinary technicians and the office workers who coordinate everything from the scheduling to the billing. Without this team work, a veterinarian would probably not be able to expand the clinic to help larger numbers of people and pets. The veterinary technicians and employees are an integral part of the interaction between the veterinarian and the pet owner. Oftentimes, they are the first and last ones to deal with worried pet owners. As such, what they say may leave a longlasting impression in the customer's mind. That's why a book such as this can be so useful, for it helps the veterinary technicians and clinic employees perceive complex medical problems in easy to understand language, so they can better grasp the pet's problems and the doctor's instructions.

### Pet Owners and Pet Fanciers

You are the ones who benefit most from the joys and beauty of pet ownership. This book was written for you. It is the hope of every contributing writer that the diseases described within these pages never affect your pets. But in the unfortunate event that your pet does suffer from a skin disorder, this book can help you better understand exactly what it is you and your veterinarian are trying to deal with. This knowledge will help you become a partner to your veterinarian, as together you work to bring health and comfort to your ailing canine or feline companion. The best general textbook for the profession remains: *Small Animal Dermatology*, published by Saunders. Let us hope that it is a work with which your veterinarian is very familiar.

*Dr. Steven A. Melman, DermaPet Inc., Potomac, Maryland*

# Acknowledgements

*Skin Diseases of Dogs and Cats: A Guide for Pet Owners and Professionals,* was written by some of the world's leading experts in the field of veterinary dermatology. These renowned professionals, who are on the cutting edge of veterinary dermatology, have written on the skin ailments and problems they know best through their research and clinical experience. And to make sure their writings remained within the grasp of pet owners who may not have any background in veterinary medicine, each chapter was carefully reviewed by some of the top editors of pet-related magazines in the United States.

I am grateful to all those who aided me in my training, and to my colleagues who provided me with the papers to complete this text. There are so many that I should thank. Specifically I want to thank my father, Dr. Harold Melman, one of the pioneers of modern veterinary practice, and Dr. Robert Schwartzman of the University of Pennsylvania, who originally inspired my dermatology training. And my thanks go out to Dr. Karen Campbell, who I had the privilege of studying with during my training, and my preceptor Dr. Erwin Small, both of the University of Illinois. Dr. Small is the motivator who inspires so many of us in this profession and made it possible for me to train in dermatology. I had the privilege of studying histopathology at the Armed Forces Institute of Pathology, Division of Veterinary Pathology, which is an unheralded group of international experts of which Major Bruce Williams, who wrote the section on Tumors, is Chief of the Training Branch. I also owe a special remembrance to my late first cousin, Dr. Greg Kedan, who helped motivate me to train in dermatology.

The colleagues who provided papers for this book are for the most part not only experts in dermatology, but also experts in the area for which they have written. For example, using the first four chapters as an illustration:

Dr. Robert Dunstan of Michigan State University, who wrote about Structure and Function, is recognized by most as one of the top five veterinary dermatopathologists in the world;

Dr. Laura Bucklan of Oradell (NJ) Animal Hospital, who wrote about Diagnostic Procedures, works in one of the largest and most respected privately owned general veterinary practices in the United States;

Dr. Alice Jeromin of the Veterinary Specialty Clinic in Richfield, OH, who wrote the chapter on Pharmacology, is a dermatology referral practitioner who also has post graduate training in the field of pharmacology.

As for my credentials, I operate the the Animal Dermatology Clinics of Potomac, MD, and Palm Springs, CA. I also founded DermaPet Inc., manufacturer of various veterinary dermatological shampoos, vitamins, food supplements and conditioners, of Potomac, Maryland.

## Special Thanks To...

**The Editors**. I want to offer special thanks to Timothy R. Fox, Managing Editor of *The Pet Dealer* magazine, who was the main editor of this book. His patience, easy-going attitude, sense-of-humor and dedication is reflected on every page. Without him it would not have been possible to translate the many professional renditions of complex diseases and treatments into a language and style that is understandable, readable and even, if possible, enjoyable. Two other renegades from *The Pet Dealer* also deserve a good deal of thanks: Paul Bubny for his editorial assistance, and Robert Conte who oversaw the artistic layout and production of this book from front to back. I am also grateful for Karen MacLeod of *Groom & Board* magazine, and John Chadwell of *Fancy Publications*, for contributing their editorial skills, and to Raymond Mensah for his keyboarding assistance. And a whole lot of thanks to Corinne Pouliquen and Kathryn Presley, for coordinating all those papers, faxes and phone calls, and to Ron Brobst, my capable veterinary technician of the last 10 years, who assisited in proofreading.

**Groomers and Pet Stylists**. I want to thank some of the people that I see as champions in the pet industry: Pam Lauritzen, founder of the International Society of Pet Cosmetologists, who runs grooming industry educational seminars, certification programs, contests and shows; Jeff Reynolds and Shirley McBride of the National Dog Groomers Association; Mario DiFante, my good friend and an international expert in grooming who runs Groom America Seminars across the country; Sally Liddick of Barkleigh Publications, who puts together *Groomer-to-Groomer* magazine and three excellent Groom Expo trade shows; Shirley and Larry Kalstone who have written books and organize the annual Intergoom event in New Jersey; and Tim Wray and Dory King of the Maryland School of Dog Grooming. Others of you that I have not named know who you are; please keep up the good work.

Groomers, you have my applause. It is you who daily deal with the skin and coat problems of our nation's pets. Sometimes I meet people who have the false impression that groomers are nothing more than pet barbers. I make it my responsibility to help people understand that your knowledge of the application and effects of shampoo on the skin is superior even to some veterinarians — although the ability to select the appropriate shampoo still remains within the veterinarian's domain!

**Kennel Operators**. You are the "innkeepers" to our nation's pets, providing a home away from home and making pet ownership more appealing — indeed, possible — to thousands of Americans. Because my brother currently operates a kennel, I've witnessed firsthand the challenges kennel operators face every day. And so I am able to applaud The American Boarding Kennel Association for its efforts in bringing kennel operators together for better cooperation and communication, and for establishing the on-going continuing education program so many years ago.

*Dr. Steven A. Melman, DermaPet Inc., Potomac, Maryland*

# Contributors

**Lowell Ackerman** DVM, HC3 Box 672 N, Payson, AZ 85541, *Nutritional Diseases, Natural Remedies*

**Al Becker** DVM, 322 Frontage Rd., Northfield, IL 60093, *Acquired Alopecia*

**Laura Bucklan** DVM, Oradell Animal Hospital, 481 Kindermack Rd, Oradell, NJ 07649, *Diagnostic Procedures, the Exam Room and Laboratory Testing*

**Kevin Byrne** DVM University of Illinois, Dept. Veterinary Clinical Medicine, 1008 W. Hazelwood Dr., Urbana, IL 61801, *Immunlogic Diseases: Food Allergy*

**Robert Dunstan** DVM, Michigan State University, East Lansing, MI 48824, *Anatomy (Structure), Physiology (Function) and Pathology of Skin*

**Dunbar Gram** DVM, Animal Allergy & Dermatology PC Hampton Roads & Richmond, 5265 Providence Road #300, Virginia Beach, VA 23464, *Diseases of Keratinization*

**Bruce Hansen** DVM, Dermatology & Allergy for Animals, 6651-F Backlick Rd., Springfield, VA 22150, *Immunologic Diseases: Overview, Laboratory Testing, Allergy Testing (In-vitro vs IDST)*

**Ann Hargis** DVM, MS, DermatoDiagnostics, 17905 Talbot Rd., Edmonds, WA 98206, *Pediatric, Congenital and Hereditary Diseases: Dermatomyositis*

**Thomas Janik** DVM, Chicago Pet Clinic, 3510 N. Cicero Ave., Chicago, IL 60641, *Hormones: The Adrenals: Hyperadrenocorticism, Corticosteroid Usage and Abuses*

**Alice Jeromin** DVM, 2785 W. Central Ave., Toledo, OH 43606, *Pharmacology and Therapeutics*

**Randy Lynn** DVM,MS, 5402 Ashbey Lane, Summerfield, NC 27358, *Pediatric, Congenital and Hereditary Diseases*

**Bill McDougal** DVM, Veterinary Allergy and Dermatology Referral Clinic, 5860 Westward Ave., Houston, TX 77081, *Eyelids, Pododermatitis and Anal Sacs*

**Patrick McKeever** DVM, University of Minnesota, C342 Veterinary Hospital, St. Paul, MN 55108, *Environmental Diseases: Burns, Frostbite and Miscellaneous Causes of Sloughing of Extremities*

**Linda Medlau** DVM, MS, Department of Small Animal Medicine, College of Veterinary Medicine, University of Georgia, Athens, GA 30602, *Fungal Diseases: Dermatophytosis (Ringworm), Ectoparasites: Demodex*

**Steven Melman** VMD, Animal Dermatology Clinic, DermaPet Inc., P.O.Box 59713, Potomac, MD 20859 *Viral Skin Diseases, Fungal Diseases: Sprortrichosis, Ectoparasites, Scabies, Flea Control, Cheyletiella (Walking Dandruff), Immunologic Diseases: Allergy, Atopy, Type I Hypersensitivity, Type 4 Hypersensitivity, Contact Allergy and Irritant Contact Dermatitis, Shar-peis and Skin Disease, Shampoo Therapy, Sebaceous Adenitis, Psychogenic Dermatoses, Ear Diseases, Eosinophilic Granuloma Complex and Miliary Dermatitis*

**Alan Mundell** DVM, Veterinary Hospital Anumal Dermatology Service, 6525 15th Ave., NW, Seattle, WA 98117, *Bacterial Skin Infections: Mycobacterium and Leprosy*

**Michael Shipstone** BVSc, Albert Animal Hospital, 3331 Pacific Hwy, Springwood, Queensland 4127, Australia, *Fungal Diseases: Cutaneous Malassezia (yeast)*

**Robert Schwartzman** DVM, School of Veterinary Medicine, University of Pennsylvania, 3800 Spruce St., Philadelphia, PA 19106, *Immunologic Diseases: Overview, Laboratory Testing, Allergy Testing (In-vitro vs IDST)*

**Margaret Swartout** DVM, Veterinary Specialty Consultation Service, Inc., 1501 Bob Kirby Rd., Knoxville TN, 37931, *Bacterial Skin Infections: Pyoderma and Immunomodulation*

**Margreet Vroom** DVM, Veterinaire Specialisten Oisterwyle Boxtelsebaan 6, 5061 VD Oisterwijk, The Netherlands, *Miscellaneous Diseases: West Highland Whites*

**Alexander Werner** DVM, Animal Dermatology Centers, 14120 Ventura Blvd, Suite K, Sherman Oaks, CA 91423, *Immunologic Diseases: AutoImmune and Immune Mediated Diseases and Immunotherapy*

**Maj. Bruce Williams** DVM, Armed Forces Institute of Pathology, Washington, D.C., *Tumors*

**Yasuyo Yamazaki** DVM, Veterinary Center for Skin Disorders, 820 Ogden Ave., Lisle, IL 60532 Chicago, IL, *Environmental Diseases: Pressure Sores, Callus, Elbow Hygroma and Photodermatitis*

**Antony Yu** DVM, Department of Small Animal Surgery & Medicine, College of Veterinary Medicine, Auburn University, Auburn, AL 36849, *Hormones: Overview, Thyroid, Growth and Sex*

# 1

# ANATOMY AND PHYSIOLOGY: STRUCTURE AND FUNCTION OF SKIN

*By Dr. Robert W. Dunstan, East Lansing, Michigan*

Anumber of years ago, I was given a young Beagle that had been born with an inability to grow hair. With the exception of short, twisted "whiskers" on its muzzle, the dog was completely bare. During its life, I was fascinated to see how my friends would respond when they handled "Lucky." Most would immediately pull their hands away at first contact, as Lucky's skin felt cool and a little moist. In short, it felt a little too "human" for comfort. Most simply said Lucky felt "disgusting." When a dog or cat has a hair coat which is not enjoyable to touch, there is a severing of the animal-human bond and your pet's value as a companion is markedly diminished. This is why there are individuals whose careers are built around grooming and bathing pets; this is why there are so many different animal skin care products; this is why skin diseases are so tragic.

All veterinarians have had dogs and cats with disfiguring skin diseases brought into their hospitals by emotionally shaken owners who may have spent thousands of dollars over several years to cure the incurable, and now want their otherwise healthy pets put to sleep. Considering the role that skin plays in the animal-human bond, and the amount of money that owners of dogs and cats spend to keep their animals' coats looking and feeling good, it is important that we have a better understanding of the *structure* and *function* of the skin of our pets.

# Overview

When most owners think of the skin of their dog or cat, they only consider its fur; however, beneath all that hair lies an organ as important for sustaining life as the heart. In its simplest terms, the skin consists of three major zones:

1) an outer layer known as the *epidermis*;

2) the *dermis*, which lies immediately beneath the epidermis; and

3) a zone composed primarily of fat and, to a lesser extent, muscle, known as the *panniculus*.

Collectively, the epidermis and dermis comprise the *cutis* and, as one could surmise, the panniculus is often referred to as the *subcutis* (Fig 1.1). Growing from the epidermis into the dermis are the *hair follicles* with their attached *sebaceous* and *apocrine* (sweat) glands (Fig 1.2). The foot pads also have glands known as *eccrine glands*, which differ from the glands of haired skin because they are not attached to hair follicles.

## The Epidermis

Even considering all its components, the skin still appears to be relatively simple; however, consider that it is the major organ which shields your pet from the external environment, and it does this through the use

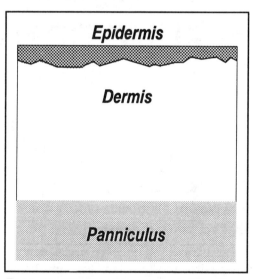

Fig 1.1 *Overview of the major components of the skin. The epidermis and dermis comprise the cutis. The panniculus is often called the subcutaneous fat.*

of many intricate mechanisms. Surprisingly, all of the major protective shields (or barriers) are present in the relatively thin epidermis. For this reason, we will begin our discussion by looking at this portion of the skin.

The epidermis is composed primarily of cells known as *keratinocytes* which are characterized by being spot-welded together at junctions known as *desmosomes*. The cells at the bottom of the epidermis (closest to the dermis) form the *basal cell layer*. This layer helps to connect the epidermis to the dermis and is composed of the only cells which normally are capable of dividing to produce the cells above them. As the cells of the epidermis grow upward, they lose their nuclei (the round central regions of cells which control every aspect of

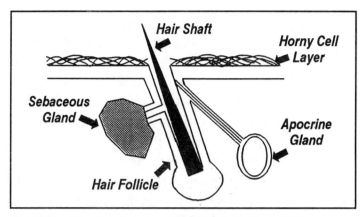

Fig 1.2 *The major adnexal structures of the skin consist of the hair follicle and attached apocrine and sebaceous glands. This diagram only shows a single hair shaft in the hair follicle. In dogs and cats many hair shafts exit through the opening of the hair follicle.*

their existence), and become elongate. Whereas basal cells have the shape of a cube or cylinder, the cells of the upper portion of the epidermis are shaped like pancakes stacked on top of each other. This layer is known as the *horny cell layer* because it is tough and composed of the same material as the horn of a cow (Fig 1.3). What makes this layer so strong is that each of these "pancakes" consists primarily of tough fibrous proteins known as *keratins*, and between these cells are fats which act as a glue holding them together. The horny cell layer makes up the major structural barrier of the skin.

In its simplest conception, your pet is surrounded by an invisible protective barrier not unlike cellophane. Nothing penetrates the horny cell layer easily from the outside or from the inside. Similarly, when this microscopic layer is lost, there is little to protect poisons or harmful organisms from entering into your pet's body, and little to prevent life-sustaining body fluids from being lost externally. Fortunately, the skin is able to rapidly replace the epidermis and its horny cell layer; however, when large portions of the epidermis are destroyed, such as occurs in severe burns, the damage can be life-threatening due to dehydration and infections.

Two other points need to be made about the epidermis and

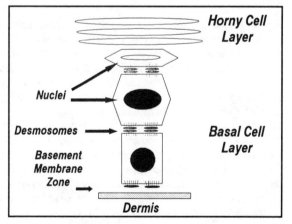

Fig 1.3 *A more detailed view of the epidermis. The cells of the epidermis move upward as they mature, becoming more elongate and eventually losing their nuclei. These anucleate cells form the major structural barrier protecting an animal's skin from the external environment. This diagram is not drawn to scale as one cell in the horny cell layer can cover 20 basal cells.*

the structural barrier of the skin. The first is that the epidermis is capable of responding to repeated injury in a dramatic fashion by becoming thicker both in the nucleated regions and the horny cell layer. Dogs or cats that continually scratch their skin have areas in which the normally smooth, supple epidermis soon resembles the bark of a tree. Such skin looks terrible, but you need to realize that just as calluses form on the traumatized skin of your hard-working hands, the thickened epidermis of a dog is a protective measure that enables their skin to better withstand repeated injury. There are a number of treatments available to diminish the thickness of the traumatized epidermis, but to use such treatments without first eliminating the cause of the scratching is analogous to treating a symptom without treating the disease. In the end, it may actually be harmful to your pet. The second point to be made is that the glue which holds the cells of the *stratum corneum* together is not a "Super Glue." Rather, it is like the glue kindergartners use: After a while, it breaks down. In normal skin, the cells in the outer portion of the horny cell layer break off in small invisible flakes as new cells replace them. In a number of skin diseases of animals, such as in seborrhea or one of a number of endocrine abnormalities, the flakes are large, not unlike dandruff in humans. These large flakes of the horny cell layer are known as *scales* (Fig 1.4). Because dogs and cats are so heavily haired, the scales often stick in the coat. These can be removed with specially formulated

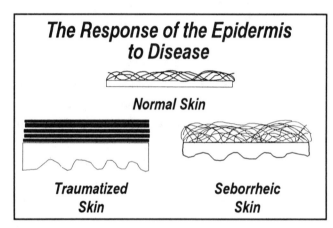

**The Response of the Epidermis to Disease**

**Normal Skin**

**Traumatized Skin**          **Seborrheic Skin**

*Fig 1.4 The normal appearance of the epidermis can change dramatically in response to trauma (i.e., itching) or other diseases such as seborrhea. Scratching is an example of an "outside-in" disease, meaning the lesions are caused by an injury that starts in the horny cell layer. In these diseases, the epidermis becomes markedly thickened. In addition, the horny cell layer, normally organized in a "basketweave" pattern, becomes laminated or compact. Clinically, such dogs have skin which is roughened and may look like the bark of a tree. Seborrhea is a disease of dogs, and less commonly, cats, in which there is excess production of a horny cell layer. In seborrhea, the horny cell layer is arranged in a normal "basketweave" pattern with only mild thickening of the nucleated layers. It is an example of an "inside-out" disease, meaning the disease is due to a primary abnormality in the basal cell layer and not injury to the horny cell layer. In contrast to trauma-induced lesions, dogs with seborrhea have excessive "dandruff" or scales.*

shampoos; however, treating a dog with severe scaliness without treating the cause is also an example of treating a symptom but not the disease, and every effort should be made to diagnose why the scales are forming.

The next major protective barrier is the immunologic barrier. Your pet is constantly being exposed to potentially harmful organisms which, if they can pass through a break in the horny cell layer, are capable of inciting an infection.

Much of the skin's ability to control infection is due to the action of *langerhans cells*. Under the microscope, langerhans cells look like an octopus, with long "arms" that extend between the keratinocytes — forming an interconnecting web with adjacent langerhans cells (Fig 1.5). The function of these cells is to take small bits of protein (known collectively as *antigens*) from whatever penetrates through the horny cell layer (be it a virus, a bacterium, a fungus or a grain of pollen) and give it to a particular type of white blood cell known as a *lymphocyte*. This results in the activation of a cascade of events which ultimately allows other white blood cells to ingest and destroy the pathogens. Nor-

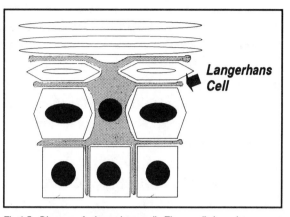

Fig 1.5  Diagram of a langerhans cell. These cells have long cytoplasmic arms forming a web between keratinocytes. Langerhans cells take up potentially injurious material, process it so the body's immune system can recognize it as foreign and ultimately, destroy it.

mally this is to your pet's benefit; however, the langerhans cells in some dogs and cats work too well. In these animals, exposure to foreign materials such as plants, pollens, house dust mites or, occasionally, even materials such as carpets, results in an exaggerated immunologic response, and an allergy develops. As any dog owner who has had a dog or cat with an allergy can tell you, such conditions are often extremely difficult to cure if exposure to the inciting antigen cannot be avoided. In such cases, treatment consists of inhibiting the immune system from reacting against the antigen by the use of glucocorticoids (steroids), essential fatty acids, and/or hyposensitization (allergy shots).

The last major barrier of the skin is the *photoprotective barrier*. Although life on earth would be impossible without the sun and the ultraviolet light it produces, for most mammals, exposing the skin to sunlight for long periods of time is very harmful. Because dogs and cats were at one time wild and lived outside all the time, they had to evolve mechanisms to protect themselves from these harmful effects. The most important photoprotective barrier in the skin of animals is the hair coat. The fur of mammals prevents ultraviolet light from coming in contact with the epidermis. As a person who is losing hair on the top of his head, I tell you firsthand how important hair is in preventing sunburn every time I am in the sun for several hours without a hat.

In addition to the hair coat, your pet has a backup photoprotective barrier in the epidermis due in large measure to *melanocytes*. These are cells interspersed between the cells of the basal cell layer which, like langerhans cells, have the conformation of an octopus. The major function of melanocytes is to produce a black or red pigment known as melanin which is packaged in granules and taken up by keratinocytes. The concentration and type of melanin produced varies from animal to animal, resulting in the variety of coat colors found in dogs and cats. When the skin or hair coat are white, the melanocytes, which are even present in non-pigmented skin, are not producing melanin. Melanin acts as a natural sunscreen which absorbs ultraviolet light and prevents it from injuring keratinocytes. In humans, who over large portions of their body have too little hair to serve as a protective barrier, there is an increase in the amount of melanin produced upon exposure to solar injury. This process, which is known as tanning, affords increased protection against sunburn. The skin of dogs and cats does not have this ability.

Occasionally, a cell in the basal cell layer which has been exposed to sunlight for long periods of time will begin to divide and grow much more rapidly than its neighboring cells, resulting in the formation of a *neoplasm* (tumor). In dogs and cats, the most common tumor which is caused by ultraviolet light is a *squamous cell carcinoma*. These tumors are malignant (meaning the tumor cells are capable of invading into deeper tissues and, occasionally, spreading through-out the body). As a rule, these tumors develop in skin exposed to sunlight where the hair is short and white. In cats, squamous cell carcinomas most commonly develop on the ears or in the skin over the bony ridges above the eyes. In dogs, these tumors occur on the abdomen (belly) of animals who spend long periods of time lying on their backs sunning themselves.

## The Dermis and Panniculus

Beneath the epidermis, surrounding the hair follicles and extending to the subcutaneous layer, is the dermis which is composed of the secretory products of cells known as *fibroblasts*: collagen, elastin and glycosaminoglycans. Although the dermis is of little importance in directly shielding the body from toxins or infectious organisms, it is essential in protecting the deeper vital organs and muscles of the body from penetrating injures. At the junction between the epidermis and the dermis is a specialized zone composed of products from the basal cells as well as collagen. This region is known as the *basement membrane* and is the site at which the basal cells and the dermis attach. There is a rare genetic disease of cats and dogs known as *epidermolysis bullosa* in which the basement membrane is defective. From birth, whenever the affected animal eats or walks, the epidermis separates from its dermal moorings. As a result, large blisters form. Most of these diseases ultimately prove fatal, testifying to how essential the basement membrane is to the function of the skin.

## Collagen

Ninety percent of the dermis consists of collagen, a strong fibrous protein which provides the tensile strength of the skin. Collagen is extremely tough and durable. Leather, the material used to make shoes, is no more than tanned dermal collagen from cattle.

## Elastin

Interspersed between the collagen bundles are structures which look similar to broken rubber bands. These are elastin fibers which, in part, provide the skin with the ability to recoil upon stretching. Although seldom identified in dogs and cats, when human skin is exposed to too much sunlight, there is an accumulation of altered elastin in the upper half of the dermis, which results in wrinkling.

## Glycosaminoglycans

The third component of the skin are the glycosaminoglycans. These are molecules which consist of chains of sugar attached to a protein core. Glyco-saminoglycans have the ability to attract a large quantity of water and maintain the normal homeostasis of the dermis. In young shar-pei dogs, dermal fibro-blasts produce excessive quantities of this material which results in the turgid texture to the skin, the "hippopotamus" appearance to the face and the many body folds.

These three components serve as a scaffold which supports the large number of vessels that provide oxygen and nutrients to the bloodless epidermis, as well as nerves which end in the epidermis and allow the animal to perceive the world around it.

## Blood Vessel Function

The dermal blood vessels play a major role in the function of the skin. First, they provide oxygen and nutrients to the epidermis as well as remove cellular wastes. Second, they play a major role in controlling your pet's body tempera-ture. You see, the skin of dogs and cats has a large number of blood vessels in the superficial dermis. Whenever your pet exercises, increased body heat is generated and there is increased blood flow to these vessels. This enables the heat to be transferred to the external environment. During cold whether the opposite occurs: The blood flow to the superficial dermal vessels is markedly diminished, thereby retaining body heat. The third major function of the dermal blood vessels is to serve as a major highway through which inflammatory cells can readily come to the skin whenever the need arises. As a result, the most common form of inflammatory skin disease is known as a *superficial perivascular dermatitis*. It is characterized by inflammatory cells surrounding the vessels of the superficial dermis.

Beneath the dermis lies the *subcutaneous fat*. It consists of lobules of fat-containing cells intersected by collagen and large blood vessels. The subcutaneous fat functions as a natural shock absorber in the skin, protecting the underlying muscle. It also functions as a nutritional "food bank," storing certain vitamins and high energy molecules known as *lipids*.

# The Adnexa

Growing from the epidermis early in the embryologic development of your pet are buds of cells from the basal cell layer which extend through the dermis. These buds eventually mature into the adnexal structures: the hair follicles with their attached sebaceous glands and apocrine glands and, in the foot pads, the eccrine glands. Because each of these structures has a different function, they will be treated individually.

### The Hair Follicles

These produce the hair shafts which make up your pet's hair coat. These hair shafts emerge through a pore in the skin. Dogs and cats have *compound* hair follicles, meaning multiple hair shafts (sometimes as many as 20) exit through each pore. This is in contrast with the skin of humans or horses and cows, which have simple hair follicles — meaning only a single hair shaft exits through each pore.

Hair has multiple functions. In addition to serving as the major photoprotective barrier, the tough keratin of which hair is composed shields the epidermis from traumatic injury. Hair also serves as "wick" by which sexually attracting chemicals produced by apocrine glands, known as pheromones, become airborne. The most important function of the hair is to control body temperature. That the hair coat would keep an animal warm in the winter should be obvious. During warm weather months, muscles attached to the hair follicle are capable of raising or lowering the hair shafts, allowing for greater or lesser circulation of air and thereby increasing or decreasing the transfer of internal heat to the external environment.

There is marked variability in the length and diameter of the hair shafts in dogs and cats. Larger hairs are known as *primary* or *guard hairs*. Smaller hairs are known as *secondary* hairs and make up the undercoat. The length of the hair shafts and the ratio of primary to secondary hairs varies from breed to breed. As a consequence, the coat of a Siberian husky has a different texture than the coat of a beagle. In addition, the hair follicles in some species are slightly twisted, resulting in hairs that are curly.

Each hair follicle goes through a cycle of active growth (the anagen stage) followed by a brief period of involution (catagen stage), ending in a period of inactivity (telogen stage) in which the old hair is shed and replaced by a new, anagen hair. The length of the anagen stage is genetically determined. In some breeds, such as German shepherds, clipping is not needed. The hair reaches a certain length and then falls out on an annual basis. Many of these breeds have a seasonal period, often in the spring, when large quantities of hair are shed. In other breeds (poodles, soft-coated Wheaten terriers, etc.) this stage may be of several years duration, and the hair is capable of growing quite long un-

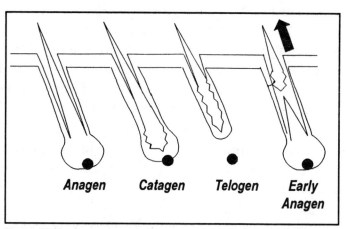

Fig 1.6 *The hair cycle. All hairs go through a cycle of active growth (anagen), shrinkage (catagen), and transient inactivity (telogen). At the beginning of the new anagen phase, the old telogen hair falls out (arrow).*

less it is clipped. Although it is often stated that these dogs do not shed, this is not true. They do shed, but to a lesser extent than most other breeds. In addition, the "non-shedding" breeds invariably have a dense coat of curly hair and the telogen hairs which fall out become enmeshed in the hair coat. Evidence of this can be found by simply brushing a "non-shedding" dog. The mounds of hair one obtains are all telogen hairs. Unless such breeds are groomed regularly, the shed hairs can form large mats which make clipping difficult and predispose the animal to developing skin infections.

In normal dogs, this cycling proceeds like clockwork. Every time a hair is lost, a new one soon replaces it. However, there are a number of diseases of both dogs and cats which are associated with *alopecia* (hair loss). Painting with a broad brush, one can categorize these diseases into 3 major categories:

1) alopecia secondary to a prolonged telogen stage;

2) alopecia secondary to pulling or plucking the hair; and

3) alopecia secondary to destruction of the hair follicle.

Alopecia secondary to a prolonged telogen stage occurs much more frequently in dogs than in cats. Almost all of these conditions are due to an underlying metabolic disease, with abnormalities of the endocrine system being most frequently implicated. In such diseases, there is either a decrease in the production of hormones necessary for hair growth or an increase in the production of hormones inhibitory to hair growth. Under either scenario, hairs enter into a prolonged telogen stage. Although the alopecia which can occur in some of these diseases can be profound, because the hairs are in a resting state, once the underlying metabolic abnormality is corrected, animals can regrow a normal hair coat.

Alopecia secondary to pulling or plucking the hair occurs much more commonly in cats than in dogs. The rough surface of a cat's tongue allows it to do its own barbering. Although self-grooming is normal in all cats, when this process becomes excessive a pattern of alopecia can develop which can appear very similar to the alopecia identified in conjunction with metabolic disease; however, microscopic examination of these traumatized hairs reveals a severed rather than a normal tapered end, and examination of a skin biopsy shows that most of the hairs are in anagen. As a consequence, once the cause of the self trauma can be eliminated (usually due to an underlying allergic skin disease) the normal hair coat will return.

Alopecia secondary to destruction of hair follicles results in a permanent hair loss. The most common cause of this condition is due to a *folliculitis* (an inflammatory reaction directed against the hair follicle) most commonly caused by either bacteria or dermatophytes (ringworm). When such a reaction is extensive, it is the most devastating of all alopecia because there is no hope for cure other than plastic surgery to replace the skin without hair follicles.

Although the diseases of the hair coat are normally associated with hair loss, owners should realize that hair is in many ways a "window into the body." In order to produce the large quantity of protein required to have a healthy hair coat, an animal must be relatively healthy. When the hair appears dry or if hair growth is slowed, even if hair loss is not present, it may be an indication of an underlying internal disease process, and it is therefore often wise to mention this to your veterinarian.

### Sebaceous Glands

These appear as foamy lobes of epithelial cells that are attached to the mid-portion of the hair follicle through a short duct. The secretion of sebaceous glands is known as *sebum* and consists of lipids (fats) and proteins. Although these glands are attached to the hair follicles of every mammal, their function remains controversial. One role is to coat, and possibly to enhance, the barrier function of the stratum corneum. Sebaceous secretions also coat the hair shafts, producing the sheen which makes the coat of a healthy dog or cat so attractive. Sebum has the ability to waterproof the skin, as evidenced in ducks, which utilize secretions of a modified sebaceous gland, the preen gland, to coat their feathers and keep them dry in water. Finally, some of the sebum's lipids keep bacteria from growing, and it has been speculated that sebum plays a role in preventing bacterial infections.

### Apocrine Glands

These are secretory organs located in the mid-to-deep dermis that are attached to the opening of the hair follicle through a long duct. In dogs and cats, apocrine glands normally secrete a viscid fluid that mixes with sebum to further seal the stratum corneum. It is also believed that some of the secretions of apocrine glands are *pheromones* — airborne hormones which function as a sexual attractant. Apocrine glands are often referred to as sweat glands. Although it may appear that this appellation is inappropriate because the normal canine and feline haired skin does not perspire (except for their foot pads, as explained in the following paragraph), in some animals with chronic skin diseases the glands of the apocrine gland will secrete a watery substance, suggesting that in certain instances, dogs and cats can perspire.

### Eccrine Glands

A modified apocrine gland, the eccrine gland is located on the pads of the feet of dogs and cats. It differs from apocrine glands in that its duct exits directly through the epidermis rather than the upper portion of the hair follicle. Also in contrast to the apocrine glands, the fluid of eccrine glands is watery and is analogous to sweat in humans. Just as a baseball player will spit on his hands to improve his grip on a bat, the major function of eccrine secretions is to increase traction.

## Summary

Treating skin diseases is different (and as a rule much more difficult) than treating diseases of any other organ system because the skin is so visible. If a dog or cat has a lung disease which responds completely to antibiotics but results in some unseen and clinically insignificant scarring of the lung tissue, most owners are content. Not so with diseases of the skin, where the demand is to have the diseased skin "look like new." In order to try to obtain this objective, treating skin diseases of animals often requires a team effort on the part of owner and veterinarian. This brief and relatively "superficial" overview of the structure and function of the skin of dogs and cats is not meant to make dermatologists out of animal owners. Rather, it should help facilitate the team effort of owner and veterinarian based on the assumption that only by understanding normal skin can pet owners comprehend what is occurring when a skin disease develops and why various treatments may be necessary.

# The Dermatology History Sheet

*The following questions are taken from actual history sheets used by many veterinarians.*

Chief complaints: _____

_____

Age and location at which the animal was purchased? _____

Has the animal been out of the area? _____
    If yes, where?   Boarding Kennel ( )   Groomer ( )   Dog Show ( )   Other ( )

Does the animal itch, scratch, bite, lick or chew? _____
    If so, when?    Constantly ( )   Sporadically ( )  Night ( )
    Where?      Feet ( )        Belly ( )        Head ( )      Back ( )
               Front Legs ( )  Back Legs ( )  Thorax ( )   Other ( )

When was the problem first noticed? _____

How old was the animal when the problem first appeared? _____

Is the problem year-round? ( ) or seasonal ( )  If seasonal, when is it worse? _____

Where on the body did the problem begin? _____

What did it look like then? _____

How has it changed or spread? _____

List any other pets: _____ Do other animals or people have any skin
    problems? _____ If so, describe: _____

When did you last see fleas? _____ Do you use insecticides in/on pet, in house
    or yard? _____ If yes, name them: _____

Describe the animal's indoor environment: _____

What percent of the animal's time is spent indoors/outdoors   _____%     _____%

Describe the animal's outdoor environment: _____

Animal's diet:
    Canned: _____  Dry: _____  Food additives: _____Other _____

What medications have been used?  List effects and dates used.
    Topical (include shampoo and conditioners): _____
    Oral: _____
    Injection: _____

Other illnesses of animal: _____

What other facts do you think would be helpful? _____

*Table 2.1*

# 2

# DIAGNOSTIC METHODS

## The Exam Room and Lab Tests

By Dr. Laura Bucklan, Oradell, New Jersey

Skin disorders are among the most common ailments that bring pets to the veterinary office, and they're perhaps one of the most difficult to diagnose. When it comes to broken bones or kidney infections, the problem can be quickly identified and isolated. But dermatological troubles present a much greater challenge, not giving themselves over to easy diagnosis. This puts the burden on the veterinarian to adopt a systematic approach when trying to uncover what is really behind all the chewing, scratching and discomfort that is common to so many skin ailments. Failure to adopt a systematic approach from the very start may lead to a series of inaccurate diagnoses and failed therapies.

## The Complete History

The first step in a systematic approach is to obtain a complete history of the patient. An accurate medical record or chart should provide much of what is needed, such as the animal's age, breed and sex. These facts can help narrow the list of possible diagnoses, since many skin problems are related to an animal's age, genetic background and gender. For example, dogs less than six months old are commonly affected with demodicosis, canine acne, juvenile pyoderma, and dermatophytosis (ringworm). Young adult and middle-aged dogs are prone to allergic disorders, hormonal abnormalities, and seborrhea. And as for the "seniors," geriatric patients are frequently affected by alopecia (hair loss) and neoplasms (tumors). Certain breeds of dogs and cats are also more prone to various skin disorders (as shown in Table 2.3, which lists some common breeds and the ailments they are predisposed to). For instance, allergic inhalant dermatitis (atopy) is common in West Highland white terriers and golden retrievers. Hypothyroidism is common in Doberman pinschers and Irish setters. In the cat world, Persians are commonly affected with dermatophytosis (ringworm).

All pet owners are expected to fully participate in helping the veterinarian gather an accurate and complete medical history. This may include filling out a history form (such as Table 2.1) that will prove invaluable to the medical expert. Questions should be answered carefully and honestly. If there is any uncertainty about something, the veterinarian should be told, because inaccurate information can be misleading. To this end, pet owners are always encouraged to keep a watchful eye on their pets, noting any unusual skin rashes and taking note of when the rash first appeared and what it looked like. If anybody other than the pet owner is responsible for bringing the animal to the veterinarian, this information should be supplied beforehand. Knowing when a skin rash first developed is important. The veterinarian will want to know whether the dog developed a rash before it began scratching and biting, or if the itching came before the rash. And what did the rash look like when it was first

## Making an Accurate Diagnosis

*In achieving an accurate dermatologic diagnosis, the veterinarian may follow these steps:*

1. History: Make note of the patient's age, breed and gender, and examine the full history of the patient's skin problems, including past and current medications.

2. Physical Examination: Identify all primary and secondary lesions, areas of hair loss, and the distribution patterns of the lesions or hair loss.

3. Initial Diagnostic and Lab Tests: Make use of routine diagnostic procedures such as skin scrapings, the Wood's light examination, bacterial and fungal cultures, and cytology. When necessary, a second array of tests may be needed, including the blood tests, hormonal assays, biopsies, allergy testing and hypoallergenic diet trials.

4. Possible Diagnoses: Using the available information, make a list of possible or differential diagnoses.

5. Narrow the List: Evaluate the information from the initial tests and examinations, and plan further diagnostic tests or therapeutic trials to narrow the list of possible diagnoses or make a definitive diagnosis.

noticed? The answers to these queries can help differentiate between allergies and other skin disorders.

You can never be too observant. It is up to you to take note of not only when the rash first appeared, but what it looked like. That's because once an animal has scratched at the rash for long periods of time, the lesions are altered and a very important clue to the problem's cause has been lost. For example, chronic allergic dermatitis and sarcoptic mange are often easily differentiated in their early stages, but once they "go chronic" they can look identical. You will also be expected to know what parts of the body are scratched or licked. Dogs with inhalant allergies will usually scratch at their face, feet, ears and axillae (armpits). Dogs with flea-bite hypersensitivity will scratch, bite and lick at their backs, tails, groins and thighs. And because certain conditions are readily transmittable to other pets, veterinarians will need to know whether or not other animals in the household are also being affected with similar conditions. The answer to this can further eliminate certain conditions from the list of possible diagnoses. For example, you may be asked if any other pets in your household have fleas. Even just a couple of fleas can be enough to cause a big problem, especially with an animal that is hypersensitive to flea bites. One bite can be enough to cause severe itching and a resulting bad rash.

Your veterinarian will also rely on you to keep track of how your pet responds to the prescribed medications. In this way, you are providing useful information to the veterinary dermatologist. It will be up to you to note whether or not any pills, injections, shampoos or topical medications have helped the skin condition. Take note of whether the medication temporarily relieved the itch but did not dispel the rash, or whether or not the problem was alleviated only to return when the medication stopped. Or perhaps the medication had little or no effect on the itch or rash. If your pet's skin problem has been going on for quite some time, or if you are being referred to a veterinary dermatologist by your regular veterinarian, it is important that you bring a copy of your pet's medical record or a letter summarizing your pet's conditions and treatments. Include the results of any tests, which will help avoid unnecessarily repeating any tests. Also bring along any medications or shampoos you are currently using or have used. With complete and accurate information, the veterinary dermatologist is best able to work towards a correct diagnosis.

## The Physical Examination

The next step in arriving at a diagnosis is the physical examination. Here the dermatologist has an advantage, since the skin can be viewed directly without the need for radiographs or scans. A thorough and systematic examination of the skin lesions, along with the medical history, can suggest the diagnosis, although tests are often needed for confirmation. The examination actually begins as soon as the patient enters the room: Does the pet lie comfortably or is the animal scratching or biting on the table? The pet should be observed from the rear, as some lesions can be as subtle as a group of raised hairs. Good lighting is essential, as is the ability to step back to observe the animal from a distance in order to determine the distribution of the lesions on the body. Observing the entire animal, the veterinarian should be able to see whether or not any hair loss is limited to one area on the body, or is it generalized? The veterinarian will also look to see whether the hair loss is symmetrical, since hair loss with bilateral symmetry may suggest a hormonal imbalance. The professional will also try to determine the general condition of the pet, seeing whether or not it is over-weight or underweight, and whether it is well-groomed or matted.

So you see, the physical exam takes in the entire animal, not just the skin. That's because *systemic diseases* can have *skin involvement*. So it is, for example, that tumors of the testicles can cause hair loss and pigment changes in the skin. And animals with diabetes will often have poor hair coat, scaly skin and superficial skin infections. This explains why the veterinarian will often start at one end of the pet and systematically examine the entire animal, including the

## *Primary Lesions*

Those lesions which develop spontaneously as a direct result of the disease. These are the most important lesions to consider when making a diagnosis.

| Lesion | Definition | Associated Diseases |
|---|---|---|
| Macule | A discreet flat spot where the skin has changed color through pigment changes, bleeding or inflammation. | Acanthosis nigricans, allergic dermatitis, bleeding disorders. |
| Papule | A small, firm elevation in the skin, often pink or red, that is caused by inflammation. | Most commonly associated with allergic disorders. |
| Nodule | A discreet, firm, solid elevation in the skin larger than 1 cm extending deeper into the skin. | Nodules are usually associated with tumors or severe inflammation. |
| Tumor | A firm swelling in the skin which may extend into the deeper subcutaneous tissue. | Benign and malignant neoplasms or cysts. |
| Pustule | A small, discreet elevation in the skin filled with pus. | Acne, folliculitis, juvenile pyoderma. |
| Wheal | A discreet, raised lesion that disappears within minutes or hours. | Hives, insect bites, positive reactions to allergy skin tests. |
| Vesicle | An elevation of the epidermis filled with clear fluid. | Autoimmune or viral disorders. |

*Table 2.2A Types of Skin Lesions*

ears, footpads and nails. It is often necessary to turn the pet over to get a closer look of the underside. You may see your veterinarian mark off the locations of lesions on a diagram of a dog or cat, which can prove helpful in monitoring ongoing changes in the condition.

With the larger examination completed, the veterinarian will then perform a closer examination of the skin itself. This may include clipping hair from a small area in order to better see and identify the lesions, which are then classified as *primary* or *secondary*:

- A primary lesion develops spontaneously and directly as a result of the disease.

- A secondary lesion results after the animal has traumatized the primary lesion with enough licking and scratching to change the original appearance.

## *Secondary Lesions*

Those lesions which derive from changes in primary lesions, such as trauma or medication. These lesions are more chronic and of a lesser diagnostic significance.

| Lesion | Definition | Associated Diseases |
|---|---|---|
| Scale | An accumulation of loose particles sloughed from the superficial layer of the skin. | Seborrhea, allergic dermatitis, demodicosis. |
| Epidermal collarette | A circular rim of scale. | Resolving folliculitis (Staphylococcal). |
| Crust | An accumulation of dried pus, blood or scale adhered to the skin and hair. | Found in many chronic dermatoses such as pyoderma. |
| Scar | An area of fibrous tissue that has replaced damaged skin and subcutaneous tissue. | Burns and deep pyoderma. |
| Ulcer | A break in the skin's surface exposing the underlying layers of the skin. | Severe pyoderma, eosinophilic ulcers in cats. |
| Excoriation | Removal of the superficial layer of skin by biting or scratching. | Acute moist dermatitis (hot spot), scabies, flea-allergic dermatitis. |
| Lichenification | Thickening and hardening of the skin, usually from friction or chronic trauma. | Acanthosis nigricans, chronic allergic dermatitis. |
| Hyperpigmentation | Darkening of the skin caused by an increase in melanin pigment in the skin. | Hormonal imbalances, any chronic dermatitis with self trauma. |
| Hyperkeratosis | An increased thickness of the horny layer of the skin, often of the footpads. | Autoimmune diseases, calluses, nasodigital hyperkeratosis (hardpad). |

*Table 2.2B Types of Skin Lesions*

A pustule is a common primary lesion, appearing as a small pus-filled blister-like elevation in the skin. Because the canine and feline epidermis is very thin, licking and scratching can easily rupture a pustule — resulting in a crust, which is then classified as a secondary lesion. Certain primary lesions are very suggestive of a specific skin disorder. However, in many cases the condition is so chronic that few if any primary lesions can be found, making it more difficult to arrive at a correct diagnosis. (Table 2.2 lists primary and secondary lesions and related possible conditions.)

The examining veterinarian will pay close attention to both the distribution of lesions and the pattern of hair loss, since these can also be very disease-specific. As with lesions, it is also possible to classify distribution patterns, although there is no need here to name them all. One worth noting by way of example, however, is the *mucocutaneous distribution pattern*, in which the lesions occur at the junction between haired skin and mucous membranes such as the lips, eyelids, anus and genitalia. A mucocutaneous distribution pattern is suggestive of an autoimmune disorder, although further testing would be necessary to confirm a diagnosis. As an example of how hair loss patterns can suggest certain ailments, there is *bilaterally symmetric* hair loss which tends to affect the trunk and spare the head and legs. Such a pattern is suggestive of a hormonal imbalance called *hyperadrenocorticism* (Cushing's Disease).

# Diagnostic Testing

It will usually be necessary to perform some sort of diagnostic test. There are a number of such tests which the veterinarian should take advantage of:

### The Skin Scraping

This simple test will likely be performed on almost every patient suffering from a skin problem, since it can help identify any microscopic parasites (such as mites) that can affect the skin. To perform a skin scraping the veterinarian needs a scalpel blade, glass slides, mineral oil, cover slips and a microscope. A drop of mineral oil placed on a glass slide is used to moisten the blade. The veterinarian will then gently squeeze the skin in order to help bring mites from their hiding places within hair follicles. This is followed by gently scraping the surface of the skin until slight bleeding occurs. The veterinarian must scrape deep enough to cause bleeding because some types of mites live deep in the skin and hair follicles. Material from the scraping is then placed on the slide, a cover slip is put on-top, and this is examined under a microscope.

A skin scraping can identify various types of mites, including *Demodex canis*, *Sarcoptes scabieii*, *Notoedres cati*, *Cheyletiella yasguri*, *Otodectes cynotis* and others.

Unfortunately for dogs suffering from scabies (sarcoptic mange), the *Sarcoptes scabieii* mites are very difficult to find on scrapings, often making it necessary to do as many as 15-20 scrapings to find even a single mite. Some animals may need sedation to allow multiple scrapings. A therapeutic trial with a miticidal preparation can be the only way to eliminate *Sarcoptes* as a possible cause for the itchy rash.

### The Wood's Light Exam

This is a useful screening test for dermatophytosis (ringworm), as well as for any unknown dermatosis. A Wood's lamp is an ultraviolet light and magnifier. Hairs that are infected with certain strains of the *Microsporum canis* fungus, a common cause of dermatophytosis in cats and dogs, will appear a fluorescent apple green when viewed with a Wood's lamp in a darkened room. Some caution is required, though, because certain medications and scaly crusty materials can appear to fluoresce. When *M. canis* is the problem, the hairs will produce the tell-tale fluorescence. However, the Wood's light exam is not the final verdict on dermatophytosis because *M. canis* will only fluoresce 50 percent of the time, and several other dermatophytes do not fluoresce at all! If no fluorescence is found, the veterinarian will likely move on to another test.

### The Fungal Culture

This test is also useful for helping determine dermatophytosis, and it involves plucking hairs from the edge of a suspect lesion and depositing them in a glass bottle or plate (such as a Petri dish) which contains a special agar solution called DTM (Dermatophyte Test Medium). The DTM agar will change from yellow to red if a fungal dermatophyte is growing on it. This test may take some time, since dermatophyte growth typically occurs between 10 to 14 days, although it may take as long as 30 days. The culture must be examined daily for growth of a fungal colony and the simultaneous color change. As an added precaution, your veterinarian may also want to culture a lesion that does fluoresce, just to confirm and identify the dermatophyte.

### The Bacterial Culture and Sensitivity Test

In some cases, a bacterial infection may be the primary cause of a skin disorder. Or else the scratching and biting that accompanies an allergic reaction may lead to traumatized skin that falls easy prey to a secondary bacterial infection. In both cases, your veterinarian may want to submit a tissue sample for a bacterial culture and sensitivity test. Because there are normally many bacteria present on the skin's surface, a meaningful culture is best taken from intact pustules using a sterile needle. If there are no suitable primary lesions available, it may be necessary to obtain tissue for culture using a biopsy instrument. Once the specimen is obtained, it will be placed in a transport media and sent to a lab that is equipped for veterinary microbiology. If bacteria are present, the lab will identify them and perform further tests in order to determine the appropriate antibiotics for treatment.

### The Cytological Examination

By studying material collected from lesions under a microscope, your veterinarian may be able to obtain a great deal of useful information. Material for the microscope can be taken from either a solid lesion (such as a nodule or tumor) or from a fluid-filled lesion (such as a pustule or abscess). This is accomplished by gently inserting a fine-gauge syringe needle into the lesion, and withdrawing the plunger several times. In most cases only a tiny drop of material will be obtained, but even this may be enough for a cytological examination. Another method for obtaining cytology material is the impression smear, in which a slide is pressed against the cut surface of an ulcerated lesion. The material is spread out into a very thin layer on a slide, and allowed to air dry before being stained. This prepared slide is then examined under a microscope by the veterinarian, or submitted to a clinical pathology laboratory. The microscopic examination may reveal the presence of various cell types and microorganisms — but not always, as some pustules may be sterile. Cell types can suggest allergy, inflammation or neoplastic (cancerous) conditions, while the presence of large numbers of bacteria or yeast organisms may also have clinical significance. The cytological examination can be especially useful when treating *otitis externa* (infection of the outer ear), which requires a sample taken from a cotton swab that has been inserted into the ear canal. The clinician will look for bacteria and/or yeast, the presence of which can lead to the selection of the right medication.

### Blood Tests

Certain cases may require blood tests, since serum chemistries and a CBC (complete blood count) are helpful in revealing underlying illnesses. For example, an increased alkaline phosphatase and certain changes in CBC can suggest hyperadrenocorticism, while a high cholesterol level is suggestive of hypothyroidism. To test for a dysfunctional thyroid, clinicians need to study the baseline levels of the thyroid hormones T3 and T4. Meanwhile, if an autoimmune disorder is suspected, blood tests such as the ANA (antinuclear antibody) may be necessary.

### Allergy Testing

If allergy is suspected as the cause of your dog's problems, the veterinarian can call upon two available testing methods: *intradermal skin testing* and *in-vitro blood testing*.

•Intradermal skin testing has been used for many years and is still considered by many the preferred method of testing. It involves clipping hair from an area on the side of the chest and using small gauge needles to inject minute amounts of various allergens (trees, grasses, weeds, molds, dust, etc.) into the skin. The injection sites are then observed for 15 to 30 minutes for signs of swelling and redness, which indicate a positive reaction. This procedure is quite painless but may require tranquilization in uncooperative patients. Certain medications such as corticosteroids (both oral and injectable), antihistamines and certain tranquilizers will interfere with the test results, which is why these drugs must be discontinued for several weeks prior to the intradermal skin test.

•In-vitro or blood tests are used to detect a certain type of antibody (IgE) in the bloodstream. The presence of the IgE antibody indicates exposure to specific allergens. These tests have the advantages of being simple to perform (simply obtain a blood sample), no hair needs to be shaved, and the animal does not have to be restrained. They are also useful if the pet's skin is so adversely affected that an appropriate area cannot be found on the body to perform intradermal skin testing.

### The Hypoallergenic/Elimination Trial Diet

If a food allergy is suspected, a hypoallergenic diet (or elimination diet) may be prescribed as a test. This involves feeding the pet a diet that includes only a single protein and carbohydrate that the animal has not yet been exposed to, such as lamb and rice. This diet must be fed exclusively for at least three to four weeks, with recent studies suggesting the feeding trial go on for as long as 12 weeks for the best results. Only after evaluating the results of such an elimination diet can food allergy be diagnosed or excluded.

### The Skin Biopsy

An extremely valuable diagnostic test, the skin biopsy is performed for a variety of reasons, such as when:

•Neither the history nor the physical examination are enough to aid a
   diagnosis;

•The lesions suggest an autoimmune or neoplastic process;

•The skin condition has failed to respond to what was thought to be
   appropriate therapy; or

•The condition looks unusual or very serious.

A biopsy should be called for whenever the veterinary diagnosis points to a serious disease that requires expensive or potentially life-threatening drugs.

# Breed Predilection for Skin Diseases

## Cats

### All breeds
Dermatophytosis (ringworm)
Eosinophilic granuloma
   complex
Ear mites
Abscess
Flea-bite allergic dermatitis
Stud tail
Acne

### Abyssinian cat
Psychogenic dermatitis
   (excessive grooming)

### Persian cat
Dermatophytosis (ringworm)
Hair mats
Facial fold dermatitis

### Siamese cat
Psychogenic dermatitis and
   alopecia

## Dogs

### Afghan hound
Hypothyroidism

### Akita
Sebaceous adenitis
Cutaneous depigmentation —
   uveitis (VKH)
Pemphigus foliaceus

### Beagle
Demodicosis
Sebaceous gland tumors

### Boston terrier
Atopy
Demodicosis

Hyperadrenocorticism
   (Cushing's Disease)

### Boxer
Acne
Atopy
Demodicosis
Hyperadrenocorticism
Neoplasma: fibroma,
   histiocytoma, mastocytoma

### Chow chow
Hypothyroidism
Pemphigus foliaceus
Hyposomatotropism (growth
   hormone responsive
   dermatosis)

### Collie
Dermatomyositis
Discoid lupus erythematosus
Nasal pyoderma

### Dachshund
Acanthosis nigricans
Demodicosis
Folliculitis
Hyperadrenocorticism
Hypothyroidism
Pattern alopecia (ears)

### Dalmatian
Atopy
Demodicosis
Folliculitis

### Doberman pinscher
Canine acne
Acral lick dermatitis (lick
   granuloma)
Color mutant alopecia
Demodicosis
Flank sucking

Folliculitis
Hypothyroidism

### English bulldog
Canine acne
Demodicosis
Facial fold dermatitis
Folliculitis
Hypothyroidism
Tail-fold dermatitis
Interdigital cysts

### German shepherd
Calcinosis circumscripta
Folliculitis and furunculosis
Discoid lupus erythematosus
Fly dermatitis of ear tips
Hemangioma and
   hemangiosarcoma
Seborrhea

### Golden retriever
Acute moist dermatitis
   (hot spots)
Atopy
Folliculitis and furunculosis
Hypothyroidism
Lymphosarcoma
Otitis externa (swimming ear)

### Great Dane
Canine acne
Acral lick dermatitis
   (lick granuloma)
Callus formation, hygroma
Demodicosis
Hypothyroidism
Pododermatitis
Folliculitis

### Irish setter
Atopy
Acral lick dermatitis
Color mutant alopecia

*Table 2.3*

Folliculitis
Hypothyroidism
Seborrhea

### Keeshond
Castration-responsive
  dermatosis
Keratoacanthoma
Hypothyroidism
Hyposomatotropism

### Labrador retriever
Acral lick dermatitis
Acute moist dermatitis (hot spots)
Atopy
Folliculitis
Lipoma
Seborrhea
Otitis externa  (swimmer's ear)

### Lhasa apso
Atopy
Hair mats

### Malamute
Zinc-responsive dermatosis
Castration-responsive
  dermatosis

### Norwegian elkhound
Keratoacanthoma
Sebaceous gland tumor

### Old English sheepdog
Demodicosis
Folliculitis

### Pekingese
Facial fold dermatitis

### Pomeranian
Hyposomatotropism

### Poodle
Epiphora (tearing)

Granulomatous
  sebaceous adenitis
Hyperadrenocorticism
  (Cushing's disease)
Hypothyroidism
Otitis externa (swimmer's ear)
Sebaceous gland tumor

### Pug
Atopy
Facial-fold dermatitis
Tail-fold dermatitis

### Rottweiler
Folliculitis
Vitiligo

### Shar-pei
Atopy
Hypothyroidism
Food allergy
Contact allergy
Demodicosis
Folliculitis
Seborrhea
Immunoglobulin A deficiency

### Schnauzer
Atopy
Hypothyroidism
Schnauzer comedones
  syndrome
Subcorneal pustular
  dermatosis

### Shetland sheepdog
Dermatomyositis
Discoid lupus erythematosus
Folliculitis
Systemic lupus erythematosus

### Siberian husky
Castration-responsive
  dermatosis

Discoid lupus erythematosus
Eosinophilic granuloma
Zinc-responsive dermatosis
Post-clip alopecia

### Cocker and Springer spaniels
Hypothyroidism
Lichenoid psoriasiform
  dermatosis
Lip-fold dermatitis
Otitis externa
Papilloma
Seborrhea

### Cairn terrier
Atopy

### Scottish terrier
Atopy
Folliculitis

### West Highland white terrier
Atopy
Seborrhea
Epidermal dysplasia
Food allergy
Otitis externa (swimmer's ear)
Cutaneous yeast

### Wire-haired fox terrier
Atopy
Sebaceous gland tumor

### Viszla
Granulomatous sebaceous
  adenitis

### Weimaraner
Lipoma
Sterile pyogranulomatous
  syndrome

That's especially true when the veterinary dermatologist's strong suspicion is based solely on an animal's medical history and physical exam. A biopsy is obtained using a biopsy punch instrument or through surgical excision with a scalpel. For most lesions, several punch biopsy specimens are adequate. If the patient is cooperative, the biopsy can be performed with local anesthesia. However, tranquilization may be called for if the lesions targeted for biopsy are on the face or feet. The specimens should be placed in formalin for transport to a veterinary pathologist (some pathologists have a special interest in dermatology) who will examine the microscopic changes in the skin and surrounding tissues. Biopsies may not always provide a definitive diagnosis, but they usually uncover some important information. For example, the biopsy can often determine if hair loss is being caused by an endocrine or hormonal imbalance, but it will not determine exactly which hormone is at fault.

## The Therapeutic Trial

If other tests have been performed with negative results, the veterinarian can make use of the therapeutic trial to pin down a strong suspicion. For example, your veterinarian may believe scabies is to blame for your dog's symptoms, but no mites turned up in the skin scraping. As a backup test, your veterinarian will try a therapeutic trial with a miticidal dip. Improvement after several such dips helps demonstrate that your veterinarian's original suspicion was correct. However, if the dips do not alleviate the symptoms, other causes must be looked for. Sometimes an animal may have more than one problem at the same time, such as an allergic inhalant dermatitis and a secondary bacterial infection. In such cases, a therapeutic trial with antibiotics can eliminate the secondary infection, making the primary problem more apparent.

# 3

# PHARMACOLOGY AND THERAPEUTICS

*By Dr. Alice M. Jeromin, Toledo, Ohio*

**M**ost people seem to think that biologically, drugs act differently in animals than they do in humans. But any student of pharmacology (the study of how drugs behave in the body) will know better. You see, although there are always differences and exceptions to the rule, by and large all species — both animal and human — show the same absorption, distribution, metabolism and excretion phases of a drug. That's because animals possess the same organs, which do the same work of absorbing, distributing, processing and eliminating medications. So really, you are not so different biologically from the cat curled up on your lap, or the dog seated at your feet. What differences there are between you and your pet are in the times that it takes drugs to be processed and eliminated (half-life), and how the body activates or inactivates the substances for its use (metabolism). Within the animal kingdom, these differences can exist between species (for example, cats metabolize aspirin much more slowly than dogs do), or within species (greyhounds are very sensitive to the barbiturate anesthetics because of their lack of body fat).

Any discussion of pharmacology should begin with the four major steps that go into the body's processing of a drug: absorption, distribution, metabolism and excretion. These apply equally to both humans and animals.

## *Absorption*

Absorption refers to the passage of an orally administered drug through the stomach or intestinal wall into the bloodstream. Food within the stomach can either help or hinder absorption. For example, the antibiotic oxacillin is best absorbed on an empty stomach, while the antifungal griseofulvin is best absorbed with a small amount of fat, such as butter or grease. It is a good idea to ask your veterinarian for any suggestions on what will help the absorption of prescribed oral medications. Injectable drugs do not rely on stomach absorption, since they are administered into the vein (intravenous), muscle (intramuscular) or under the skin (subcutaneous). This allows the drug to enter the system much more quickly, but it does have the disadvantage of being "past the point of no return." At least an orally administered drug can be vomited up, if necessary, before it is absorbed.

### Distribution

Distribution refers to the body tissues (mainly water- or fat-cells) that absorb the drug after it passes from the stomach or intestine. A good deal depends on the amount of blood flow to that affected area, the amount of lipid (fat) present, or the acidity of the drug. Some drugs need to "pair up" with a protein (protein-binding) in order to do their work, while others will combine with a particular receptor located on the outside of a cell in order to gain entrance into the cell.

Other drugs such as barbiturates (phenobarbital) will be stored in body fat reservoirs. Because fat has little blood flow, drugs stored in fat tend to remain in the body longer.

### Metabolism

Metabolism, or *biotransformation*, usually occurs within the liver, and serves to deactivate (or, in some cases, activate) a drug. For example, there are special enzymes in the liver that can detoxify potent drugs, which are then eliminated from the body. Species differences can determine which enzymes are present. For instance, cats do not have glucuronide enzymes, which serve to detoxify aspirin. In young animals, including humans, some liver enzymes are not fully developed, which means that giving an infant certain drugs (such as chloramphenicol) can be like providing a poison pill rather than a medical cure. Because of the liver's importance, animals with impaired liver functioning should receive only those drugs that do not pass through this detoxifying organ. Otherwise, drugs that require liver clearance should only be administered in smaller doses.

### Excretion

Excretion of most drugs takes place through the kidney, a complex organ consisting of tubules which filter out and/or reabsorb substances. Drugs are excreted as detoxified substances (metabolites) or unchanged. The pH of the drug is significant, since acidic drugs are excreted more rapidly in a basic (alkaline) urine, and vice versa. This information is important when treating poisonings, since knowing the acidity or alkalinity of a drug can determine whether or not the urine should be made more acidic or basic to speed the process of elimination. Because kidney function (renal function) slows down as an animal ages, it is important when working with older animals to reduce the dose of medications which are eliminated by the kidney. If this is not taken into consideration, toxicities can occur. An example is the antibiotic gentamicin. It is actually possible to measure levels of gentamicin in the body to determine that a destructive toxic level will not be reached in the kidneys.

## Drugs and Dermatology

Although a plethora of drugs exist in veterinary medicine, this chapter will concentrate most heavily on those used most often in veterinary dermatology. Unfortunately, it is impossible in one short chapter to list all the side-effects associated with a medication. However, I have listed those seen most frequently in practice, along with "textbook" reports. General doses are included, but remember: Always follow your veterinarian's directions to the letter. And make sure you understand why your pet is being given a certain medication, and the potential for side-effects that may be encountered. More importantly, do not administer over-the-counter human drugs to your pet without checking first with your veterinarian. If at any time you feel your pet is experiencing an adverse reaction from any medication, alert your veterinarian!

## Antihistamines

Perhaps the most frequent complaint of people whose pets have allergic skin diseases is the amount of scratching the animals go through. Although in many instances the itching is relieved by cortisone, most pet owners are aware of the numerous side-effects associated with cortisone and prefer to avoid it. To try to give the pet (and the owner!) some relief, veterinarians may prescribe other medications, such as antihistamines, which are commonly used for people with allergies. When an animal is exposed to an allergic substance (an allergen) by either touching or inhaling it, certain chemicals are released in the animal's body. These chemicals include histamine, prostaglandins, leukotrienes, thromboxanes, to name a few. These chemicals cause changes in the blood vessels, building up to inflammation.

When this occurs in humans, we refer to it as hayfever — with all its accompanying symptoms of runny nose and itchy eyes. Well, the same process occurs in animals, except that rather than wheeze and sneeze, animals tend to itch and scratch — especially their faces and feet. Drugs such as antihistamines are used to block the release of the inflammatory chemicals, thereby preventing the subsequent inflammation and itching. The problem with using antihistamines in veterinary medicine is that at best, only one out of five dogs will have their symptoms relieved. This is probably because histamine is only one out of many chemicals (discussed above) that is released during an allergic attack. However, because antihistamines have very few side-effects in animals, veterinarians will frequently prescribe these drugs for allergic animals with a hope for their effectiveness. If the prescribed antihistamine is not effective, the veterinarian may switch the pet to another after a week or so, since there are many antihistamines on the market — each being slightly different chemically from the other.

There are generally few side-effects of antihistamines, with the main problem being sleepiness. This usually lasts only a few days, but if it continues beyond that the dosage should be lowered. As a group, antihistamines should be used cautiously in dogs with epilepsy (they may promote seizures), glaucoma and heart problems. Antihistamines may also lead to dryness of the mouth and/or constipation. Occasionally, antihistamines — particularly chlorpheniramine — may cause increased itching and hyperexcitability. Most antihistamines should

## *Antihistamines Used in Veterinary Medicine*

| Brand Name | Generic Name | Rx Needed | Oral Dose** |
|---|---|---|---|
| Atarax[1] | hydroxyzine | yes | 1 mg/lb b-tid* dog & cat |
| Benadryl[2] | diphenhydramine | no | 1 mg/lb b-tid dog |
| Chlortrimeton[3] | chlorpheniramine | no | 2-12 mg b-tid dog<br>2-4 mg bid cat |
| Seldane[4] | terfenadine | no | 2.5-5 mg/lb bid dog |
| Tavist[5] | clemastine | no | 1.34 mg bid dogs<30 lbs.<br>2.68 mg bid dogs>40 lbs. |
| Temaril[6] | trimeprazine | yes | 0.5-1 mg/lb tid dog |

**I would start at the lower end of the dosage if buying these over the counter. If prescribed by the clinic, follow the veterinarian's instructions.

*bid = 2x daily, tid= 3x daily

[1]Atarax, Roerig    [2]Benadryl, Parke-Davis    [3]Chlortrimeton, Schering    [4]Seldane, Marion Merrill Dow
[5]Tavist, Sandoz    [6]Temaril, Herbert

Table 3.1

not be used in pregnant animals. Research in human medicine has recently led to an advisory against the combined use of the antifungal drug ketoconazole (Nizoral, Janssen) or the antibiotic, erythromycin, with terfenadine (Seldane, Marion Merrell Dow) because of the side-effect of an irregular heart rate. Although this has not been demonstrated in animals, it is probably best to avoid using these two drugs together. For better absorption, a pet should have an empty stomach when taking antihistamines.

It is also advised that antihistamines be given *before* an allergic attack, and on a regular basis during the allergy season. A few antihistamines are available without a prescription, while the rest can be obtained through a veterinarian with a prescription.

Finally, a few words need to be said about topical antihistamines such as Benadryl[2] Cream and Histacalm shampoo. Although these may have a "calming" effect on the pet due to the soothing ingredients in the "vehicle" or carrier substance, there is no good evidence that antihistamines applied topically are effective.

## Antibiotics

The most common problem I see in my veterinary practice is a bacterial infection caused by the common *Staphylococcus* species. The infection can look different in various breeds of dogs. For example, the short-coated breeds such as the shar-pei, viszla, Dalmatian or Labrador retriever will take on a "moth-eaten" look, while long-haired breeds such as the German shepherd, Siberian husky or golden retriever will have a red, pimply rash that expands outward to form a ring-like lesion. "Hot spots," "Staph" and folliculitis are terms that refer to this canine bacterial infection.

Unfortunately for the afflicted dog, a bacterial infection is often mistaken for a seasonal allergy because it tends to occur in warm weather, when the humidity levels are high. Infection in most dogs leads to itchiness, and that, too, leads owners to believe their dogs are allergic to something. For cats, bacterial infections are less of a problem, since most felines are fastidious in their grooming habits.

Whenever I am unsure as to whether or not a dog has an allergy with an accompanying infection, or an infection with an underlying allergy, I will prescribe antibiotics and antibacterial bathing. The antibiotics are to be taken for as long as necessary until all lesions are gone. If any itching remains, the pet requires further examination for allergy. A common mistake is to administer antibiotics for only two weeks at most, after which time pet owners are requested to report back to the veterinarian. It is essential that the owner let the veterinarian know how the dog is doing during this time so that therapy can be continued until all lesions have resolved.

There are numerous antibiotics available in veterinary medicine. The following are those used most often in veterinary dermatology:

### Erythromycin

(Various manufacturers) (5-10 mg/lb bid). This antibiotic works by stopping the formation of essential proteins in the bacteria. It is inexpensive and has a low toxicity. However, bacteria can easily develop a resistance to erythromycin, making it less effective for repeated use. The main side-effect is vomiting, which means the drug should be given with a small amount of food to make it easier on the stomach. Sometimes it is administered with another drug designed to calm the stomach. An alternative is to offer erythromycin in small doses initially, then gradually working up to the full recommended dose.

### Clindamycin

(Antirobe, Upjohn) (2.5-5 mg/lb bid). This antibiotic works in the same manner as erythromycin, but without the unpleasant side-effect of vomiting. Its other advantage includes a twice-daily dosing and the ability to fight both surface- and deep-infections. However, since clindamycin and erythromycin are closely related, you can safely assume that if erythromycin is ineffective, not much can be expected of clindamycin either. A side-effect of clindamycin in humans is irreversible diarrhea or colitis, an affliction that has only rarely been seen in animals.

### Sulfonamides

(Tribrissen, Coopers; DiTrim, Syntex; Primor, Roche) (10-15 mg/lb bid dog). These antibiotics are actually a combination of a sulfa antibiotic and a non-sulfa, trimethoprim or ormetoprim. They work against bacteria by interfering with the formation of folate, which is essential for bacterial metabolism. Advantages include twice-daily dosing, and a relatively low price tag. Disadvantages include resistance when used repeatedly for a chronic infection, as well as some side-effects.

Sulfa antibiotics in general should be used cautiously in dogs with dry eye (*keratoconjunctivitis sicca*), or in breeds which are predisposed to dry eye (Lhasa apso, shih-tzu, Boston terrier, bulldog, schnauzers, Westies). Dry eye symptoms include mucous discharge from the eye, the lack of a shiny gloss to the eyeball, squinting, or rubbing of the eye. There have also been reports of seizures or odd behavior after administration of only one or two doses of sulfonamides in dogs. I do not recommend the use of sulfonamides in Doberman pinschers because of a breed-related generalized side-effect of arthritis, muscle/retinal and/or kidney inflammation, anemia and erythema multiforme (a drug reaction limited to the skin). Sulfa drugs in general should be taken with plenty of water, and used cautiously in patients with compromised kidney function because of their tendency to form crystals in the kidneys. However, urine crystallization has been reported more often in human medicine than veterinary medicine.

### Amoxicillin with clavulanic acid

(Clavamox, Beecham) (6.25 mg/lb tid). Clavamox is an effective antibiotic against *Staphylococcus*, and works by preventing formation of the bacterial cell wall. The clavulanic acid component goes against a bacterial enzyme which would normally be able to render amoxicillin useless. This antibiotic is similar to Augmentin (Beecham), which is used in humans. When dealing with animal skin infections, veterinarians should recommend a three-times daily dosing schedule. Clavamox has few side-effects, and should not be taken if the patient is allergic to penicillin.

### Oxacillin

(Bactocill, Beecham). Oxacillin works the same way as Clavamox by inhibiting bacterial cell wall formation. It is also not affected by the bacterial enzyme that neutralizes amoxicillin. Side-effects are rare, although patients allergic to penicillin should not take oxacillin. For best absorption, the drug should be taken one hour before or two hours after mealtime.

### Cephalexin

(Keflex, Dista) (10 mg/lb bid or tid); *Cephradine* (Velosef, Squibb). The name for this group of antibiotics, which includes cephalexin and cephradine, is cephalosporin. Cephalosporins work by interfering with the bacteria's ability to build its cell wall. They are particularly effective against *Staphylococcus* bacteria, and can be used in chronic infections, with resistance developing only rarely. In my practice, I have had the most success with this drug in treating chronic infections. Side-effects are few, and include loss of appetite, vomiting, lethargy and increased water consumption. Because the drug is eliminated through the kidneys, a lower dose should be used in older animals. And with penicillin-allergic animals, there is a three-to-five percent chance of the animal also being allergic to the cephalosporins, since the two are chemically similar.

### Enrofloxacin

(Baytril, Haver) (2.5 mg/lb bid dog). Enrofloxacin is a member of the quinolone group of antibiotics, which includes Cipro (Miles) used in humans.

The quinolones work by preventing bacterial DNA from replicating. An advantage is their activity against *Pseudomonas* bacteria, which can be present in deep infections and present the dermatologist with a real challenge in treatment. They are also effective against *Staphylococcus* and other bacteria, hence they are referred to as broad-spectrum antibiotics (as are Clavamox, Cephalexin and the sulfas mentioned above). They should not be used in animals less than six months of age, because of possible damage to joint cartilage. Other side-effects include a lack of appetite and vomiting, but these are rare.

### Chloramphenicol

(Chloromycetin, Parke-Davis) (20 mg/lb tid). This drug is also a broad-spectrum antibiotic that works by preventing bacterial protein synthesis. It should not be used in young animals because it is metabolized in the liver, and young animals may not yet have the enzymes necessary to break it down. It has few side-effects in dogs, but is rarely used in humans because it can lead to anemia. When handling this drug or administering it to a pet, strong precautions must be taken to avoid direct contact. Because of this potential for anemia in humans, some states ban the use of chloramphenicol completely, even with animals, if another equally effective drug is available.

> •Note: If your pet has difficulty taking tablets or capsules, ask the veterinarian for a liquid form of the antibiotic. Many of these are available in a flavored liquid that can be added to yogurt or ice cream to make the going-down more pleasant.

# Retinoids

The name "retinoids" refers to the entire group of natural and synthetic vitamin A drugs which are necessary for normal skin maturation and keratinization, as well as vision and reproduction. Vitamin A is a fat-soluble drug that is easily stored in the liver. This means it can build up to toxic levels if oversupplemented. Synthetic vitamin A derivatives such as isotretinoin (Accutane, Roche), etretinate (Tegison, Roche) and topical tretinoin (Retin-A, Ortho) were developed for use in humans to intensify the effects of vitamin A while minimizing the toxicities. Uses of retinoids in humans include acne, ichthyosis and psoriasis. In general, their effect is to normalize skin and glands in the skin that are turning over too quickly. The same mechanism of action has been used with certain skin problems in cats, dogs and even a llama!

Natural vitamin A, isotretinoin and etretinate have been used individually with success in cases of vitamin A responsive dermatosis of the American cocker

## Oral and Topical Retinoids

| Brand Name | Generic Name | Dose |
|---|---|---|
| Vitamin A (oral) | Vitamin A | 300-400 units/lb. daily or higher |
| Accutane[1] (oral) | isotretinoin | 0.5-1mg/lb. daily or higher |
| Tegison[2] (oral) | etretinate | 0.5-1mg/lb. daily or higher |
| Retin-A[3] (topical) | tretinoin | Apply sparingly once or twice daily* |

[1]*Accutane (Roche)*     [2]*Tegison (Roche)*     [3]*Retin-A (Ortho)*
*Excessive application results in a local "hypervitaminosis A" reaction consisting of redness, irritation and pain.*

Table 3.2

spaniel. While this illness primarily afflicts the cocker, it has also been reported in other breeds. Canines suffering from vitamin A responsive dermatosis are afflicted with excessive scaling that adheres to the hair, a rancid odor that even frequent bathing can't get rid of, and chronic bacterial skin infections. The disease is diagnosed by a skin biopsy (often performed by the veterinarian and sent to the dermatopathologist). In these cases, I would prescribe natural vitamin A for 60 to 90 days, and if no improvement occurs the next step would be isotretinoin or etretinate therapy (see Table 3.2).

Other uses for retinoids in veterinary medicine include ichthyosis, sebaceous adenitis, early squamous cell carcinoma, follicular dysplasia, mycosis fungoides, multiple keratoacanthomas, epidermal inclusion cysts, feline idiopathic ulcerative dermatosis and schnauzer comedo syndrome. Topical tretinoin has also been used successfully in feline chin acne and acanthosis nigricans of the Dachshund.

But still, despite all the breakthroughs, retinoids are not without their side-effects — perhaps the most important one being birth defects. Human patients must practice strict contraceptive precautions while taking the synthetic retinoids, and for some times afterwards. It is not known how long after retinoid therapy animals can be bred; one retinoid (etretinate) is deposited in fat and tends to remain in the body for a long time. Other reported veterinary side-effects include increased cholesterol and triglycerides, dry eye, joint pain or stiffness, difficulty in chewing, hyperactivity, vomiting or diarrhea. Initially I would monitor every month — via blood samples — cholesterol and triglyceride levels in patients taking retinoids. Afterwards I would monitor patients only twice yearly.

A Schirmer tear test for dry eye is performed two weeks after the start of retinoid therapy, then monthly for the first few months. I also advise the owner to watch for signs of dry eye, such as excess mucous discharge, lack of glossiness to the eyeball, and pawing or rubbing the eye. This is especially important for dogs prone to dry eye, such as Lhasa apsos, cocker spaniels and Westies. The owner must realize that in most of these diseases, retinoid therapy may not provide a cure, but it can control the disease. Owners should also be warned about the expense of the medications, although natural vitamin A is relatively inexpensive. Depending on the size of the dog, isotretinoin or etretinate therapy can run into the hundreds of dollars monthly. However, in many cases, once improvement has occurred, the dosage can be cut back to the lowest amounts needed to maintain control.

Owners must be very careful not to accidentally ingest any retinoids, given their potential side-effects.

## Corticosteroids

"Steroids," "cortisone" and "Pred" all refer to a group of drugs called corticosteroids or glucocorticoids. In this section, we will stick to the terms corticosteroids and steroids.

The corticosteroids and steroids play an essential role in the body's metabolism. They are responsible for giving the body energy by maintaining blood glucose concentrations, storing glucose in the liver for future needs, controlling potassium and sodium concentrations, and enabling us to survive "fight or flight" situations. Steroids are produced by the adrenal glands, which are located next to both kidneys. The pituitary gland in the brain sends a signal to the adrenal glands, which respond by producing cortisone. Endogenous, or "natural cortisone," is produced at approximately 0.5 mg/lb/day in dogs. In both dogs and humans, the highest secretions occur in the in the morning hours. It is hypothesized that in the cat, secretion levels are higher in the evening, given the feline's nocturnal nature.

Most exogenous (oral or injectable) steroids are used for their anti-itching or anti-inflammatory effects. However, steroids can also boast immune suppression and anti-cancer benefits. The anti-inflammatory effects of steroids are important in cases of arthritis and spinal cord trauma. They prevent inflammation by inhibiting movement of cells into the area where they could release chemicals and cause damage. Steroids are also valuable in controlling immune system diseases such as pemphigus or systemic lupus erythematosus. The drugs interfere with the body's immune response, which in lupus erythematosus can be greatly exaggerated.

Overall, steroids can be life-savers, especially in cases of shock, lymphoma and other cancers, and immune-mediated diseases such as lupus, pemphigus and bullous pemphigoid. But steroids also have a dark side. In my practice, most clients know that steroids are "bad" and want to steer clear of their use. However, they must come to understand that the designation of "bad" depends in large part upon the dose and length of time the drug is administered.

Normally, steroids given for two weeks or less at a dose of 0.25 to 0.5 mg/lb daily will not produce long-lasting side-effects — which are more likely to occur from chronic daily administration, or even chronic intermittent administration. Most owners recognize the early side-effects of steroids, including increases in drinking (polydipsia), appetite (polyphagia) and urination (polyuria). Increased panting and altered mental alertness may also occur. There are also internal changes which can affect several body systems: muscle weakness, osteoporosis, pancreatitis, stomach and intestinal ulcerations, "pot belly," increased cholesterol levels, fatty liver, diabetes, decreased thyroid levels, decreased ability to fight off infection, hair loss, thin skin, easy bruising and iatrogenic Cushing's Disease. (This latter disease is caused by an excess of

---

## *Ten Tips When Giving Steroids to Your Pet*

*If steroids are prescribed by your veterinarian, it is important to follow these suggestions:*

1. Administer the drug with food, after a full meal, if possible, to reduce the potential for gastric irritation.

2. Give the dose in the morning, if prescribed for a dog, and in the evening for a cat.

3. Never abruptly discontinue steroids. Animals need to be weaned away from the drugs slowly, over a period of weeks, especially if the steroid treatment had been over a long period of time.

4. Giving steroids every other day is preferred to daily administration because it still allows the body's adrenal glands to produce "natural cortisone." (Long-term daily use shuts off the adrenal glands' production of steroids.)

5. Any infection noticed by the owner should be brought to the veterinarian's attention.

6. The animal's stool should be watched for any black, tarry colors or signs of fresh blood. The veterinarian should be contacted immediately if either of these are present

7. Any vomiting while on steroids could be a sign of pancreatitis (inflammation of the pancreas). Some schnauzers are prone to pancreatitis by having an idiopathic hypercholesterol condition in the breed, and should be carefully observed for vomiting.

8. Thyroid levels can be artificially lowered while a dog is receiving steroids. I prefer the animal be off steroids for three months before performing a regular thyroid test (a TSH stimulation test may be more of a help).

9. Pets with heart conditions should take steroids cautiously, since they can cause sodium retention which leads to increased blood pressure and heart strain.

10. Many people do not realize that chronic steroid use will cause substantial hair loss. Steroids place the hair follicle in an arrested phase, and delay growth of replacement hair.

cortisone in the body which, when given orally, shuts off the body's natural production.) Any and all of these changes can occur particularly from long-term steroid use, and many are reversible upon discontinuation of the drug.

What is not known is how long it takes for steroids to be eliminated from the body once the drugs are discontinued, or how long till the side-effects go away. For example, it can take several months for the weight gain and pot-bellied appearance to go away.

When steroids are chosen as the treatment of choice, it is best to use a short-acting steroid such as prednisone (see Table 3.3). A short-acting steroid will not stay in the system long enough to cause adrenal suppression.

## *Characteristics of Various Glucocorticoids for Administration*[*]

| Short-Acting | Intermediate | Long-Acting |
|---|---|---|
| Hydrocortisone | Triamcinolone[4] | Flumethasone |
| Prednisolone[1] | | Dexamethasone[5] |
| Prednisone[2] | | Betamethasone |
| Methylprednisolone[3] | | |

[*]From Scott, D.W.: Dermatologic Use of Glucocorticoids; Vet. Clinic North America (Small Anim. Pract.) 11:19, 1982.

[1]Various manufacturers   [2]Various manufacturers   [3]Medrol, Upjohn   [4]Kenalog, Squibb   [5]Decadron, MSD

Table 3.3

Oral steroids are preferred over injectables, except in an emergency. An exception to this rule is the use of Depo-Medrol (Upjohn) in the cat. Because felines are generally more resistant to the effects of steroids, they are less likely than dogs to develop side-effects. Often, cats will require higher doses administered through injection. It has been hypothesized that cats have fewer numbers of the receptors which steroids bind to, lowering the binding levels for cats as compared to dogs.

Topical steroids such as those purchased over the counter (one percent hydrocortisone) or prescribed by the veterinarian such as Panalog (Solvay), Tritop (Upjohn), Lidex (Syntex), Synalar (Syntex) or Temovate (Glaxo) to name a few, also have anti-inflammatory effects. When applying any topical steroid to an animal, it is important for the owner to wear gloves or a finger cot to prevent absorption into the human system. There can be a considerable amount of systemic absorption of topically administered steroids, particularly with the most potent topicals like Temovate. Prolonged use of topical steroids can cause thinning of the skin, hair loss, scaling and the systemic side-effects mentioned in this chapter. I request that my patients use topical steroids, initially, for only two weeks. Then I have them return for a re-examination to determine if we can reduce the dose.

## Non-Steroidal Anti-Inflammatory Agents

The non-steroidal anti-inflammatory drugs (NSAIDS) are a group composed of drugs that work against inflammation without steroid activity. Therefore, they do not possess many of the undesirable side-effects seen with steroids. These drugs are used in humans for arthritis pain, muscle pain and headaches. Included in this group are the essential fatty acids, which are discussed elsewhere in this book. There are few NSAIDS used in veterinary medicine (see Table 3.4), and they are mainly used in cases of arthritis, strains and sprains. Theoretically they can inhibit mediators of inflammation (prostaglandins, thromboxanes) and have been used by some to relieve allergic symptoms. Because there are many mediators of inflammation, and NSAIDS inhibit only a few, they do not have a strong role in the veterinary treatment of allergy.

Side-effects include stomach irritation and even ulcers. All NSAIDS should be given with food, preferably after a full meal. The veterinarian should be notified if vomiting, black tarry stools or blood in the stools occur. Other potential side-effects include kidney failure and bleeding tendencies, since these drugs inhibit blood-clotting (platelet aggregation). The NSAIDS should be used carefully (if at all) in older animals or those with reduced kidney function.

Ibuprofen derivatives such as Motrin (Upjohn) or Advil (Wyeth Ayerst) should not be used in dogs and cats because of the danger of gastric ulcers and kidney failure.

## Non-Steroidal Anti-Inflammatory Drugs

| Brand Name | Generic Name | Dose |
|---|---|---|
| Ascriptin* | Aspirin | dog: 10 mg/lb 3x daily |
|  |  | cat: 10 mg/lb 2x weekly** |
| Butazolidan[1] | Phenylbutazone | dog: 6-7 mg/lb 3x daily up to 800 mg/day |
| Naprosyn[2] | Naproxen | dog: 1 mg/lb 1x daily (used cautiously) |
|  |  | cat: not recommended |

*Ascriptin (Rorer) is the preferred form of aspirin because it contains an antacid for buffering.
**Aspirin must be used with great care in cats because it tends to stay in the system a very long time.
[1](Butazolidan, Geigy)        [2](Naprosyn, Syntex)

Table 3.4

# *Shampoo Step Therapy*

Shampoo *"Step Therapy"* provides dogs with relief from almost all seborrhea, dry or scaling skin disorders, itching as resulting from atopy or contact allergies, and skin infections. Although many products can be substituted, this process was created by the author using DermaPet® products.

### *STEP ONE*

A. Apply a hypoallergenic moisturizing shampoo[1] that contains essential fatty acids. As with all shampoos, leave the suds on the lathered pet for at least 10 minutes before rinsing.

B. Apply a conditioner[2] directly to the wet coat, and allow it to dry.

C. Spray conditioner on the coat daily.

   *Note: If the problem persists or if moderate pyoderma (skin infection) is present, either on the surface or superficially, proceed to Step Two.

### *STEP TWO*

A. Repeat A from Step One to prime the coat.

B. Apply a solubilized sulfur/salicylic acid shampoo.[3] Leave the suds on the lathered pet for the required 10 minutes.

C. Repeat B and C from Step One.

   *Note: If the problem persists, if the coat is oily and/or if hot spots, skin infections, chin acne, oily skin or bad skin odors are present (or if you are bathing a West Highland white terrier or a shar-pei), then proceed to Step Three.

### *STEP THREE*

A. Repeat A and B from Step Two. Although B is optional, it may be helpful due to synergism between sulfur and benzoyl peroxide.

B. Apply benzoyl peroxide.[4] (Note: A combination Sulfur/Benzoyl Peroxide Shampoo may allow the bather to omit Step 2.) Remember to allow the suds to sit for at least 10 minutes.

C. Repeat B and C from Step One.

The merits of Step Therapy are many. The severity of the therapy will vary from case to case and according to the individual pet's needs. Combination products are "shotgun" treatments for problems that might not be serious; they can cause complications in severe cases when an animal's skin is most sensitive. The use of Step Therapy not only ensures a more benign treatment protocol, it also allows more thorough application of effective ingredients.

1. *Conditioning Shampoo[a] Mycodex HA[b] and Allergroom[c].*

2. *Conditioner[a]. For itching dogs, use Oatmeal Conditioner[a].*

3. *Seborrheic[a] or Sebolux[c].*

4. *Benzoyl Peroxide[a], Mycodex BP[b]. Step Two can be skipped with Benzoyl Peroxide Plus[a] or Sulfoxidex[d].*

   *a. DermaPet    b. SmithKline Beecham and Norden    c. Allerderm/Virbac    d. DVM*

# 4

# SHAMPOO THERAPY

*The following is based on articles appearing in The Pet Dealer (October, 1992), Groom and Board (July, 1993) and Vet Forum (March and May, 1993)*

*By Dr. Steven A. Melman, Potomac, Maryland*

Of the approximately 116 million dogs and cats in the United States, anywhere from 12 to 20 percent suffer from allergy-induced skin problems. At one time, veterinarians used to rely quite heavily upon drugs to bring relief and healing to these ailing housepets. But today, the veterinary establishment has come to appreciate the importance of frequent bathing and the use of "hypoallergenic" shampoos as a way of speeding animals towards recovery. Known as "shampoo therapy," this relatively new method of treatment involves the use of cleansing, moisturizing, anti-seborrheic, degreasing, anti-parasitic, anti-bacterial, anti-fungal and anti-pruritic (anti-itch) shampoos.

Veterinarians will select a shampoo product and establish a bathing regimen according to the patients' skin characteristics, such as dryness, oiliness, scaling, inflammation and associated pyoderma (infection). (Many of these subjects are discussed in greater detail in separate sections of this book.) Generally, pet owners prefer the use of a more refined, milder product rather than a coarser, more potent one. Their hope is to reduce the risk of irritation and side effects that could possibly result from a shampoo that is too strong. But there are many more factors to consider aside from product strength or skin characteristic. This article, then, will explain various issues that need to be taken into consideration when selecting therapeutic shampoos that will relieve the various symptoms that plague our pets.

## Cleansers and Moisturizers

Cleansing and moisturizing shampoos are designed to do just what their names say. The mechanical process of bathing (even with water alone) helps remove scales, crusts, organisms, dander, loose hair and other debris. All such shampoos should be pH-adjusted for dogs, which have the highest skin pH (6.2 to 7.2) of any mammal, including humans (5.6 avg.). In addition, most good products contain essential fatty acids, which help provide nutrients to the skin. Certain vitamins such as biotin and pro-vitamin B-5 (pantothenic acid), which are said to help thicken hair, and vitamin E, which is an excellent natural antioxidant, also serve to prolong the shelf life of many shampoos. This category includes products said to be "hypoallergenic" and "all-natural." But be aware: There can be a huge difference between a product that is "all-natural," and one that is truly "hypoallergenic."

- The "all-natural" label means that none of the product's ingredients were man-made or synthesized.

- The "hypoallergenic" label means that the product should contain very few substances that could cause an allergic reaction. Hypoallergenic shampoos should be the least irritating products on the market.

That's why you should never confuse one for the other, because some "all-natural" shampoos may contain colorants, whiteners, deodorants, and added colors or fragrances that can be potent irritants and sensitizers for allergies. Even some natural ingredients such as oatmeal, aloe vera, melaleuca oil, tea tree oil, citrus extracts and eucalyptus may be primary irritants or allergens. In fact,

## Animal vs. Human Skin

|  | Cat/Dog Skin | Human Skin |
|---|---|---|
| **Type of Follicle** | Compound: Many hairs per pore | Simple: One hair per pore |
| **pH** | 6.2 pH to 7.2 pH<br>Average: 6.6 pH | 5.2 pH to 6.2 pH<br>Average: 5.6 pH |
| **Epidermal Thickness** | Thin: 4 to 6 cell layers | Thick: 8 to 12 layers |
| **Sweat Glands** | Only in foot pads, bridge of nose | Throughout the body |
| **Sebaceous Glands** | All over the body | Predominant in face, hairy areas |
| **Epidermal Transit Time (from formation to shedding)** | 22 days | 28 days |

Table 4.1

d-limonene — a well-known natural citrus extract used as a pesticide in many formulations — was used in World War II as a de-greaser on war ships! Other natural ingredients which are used for their moisturizing and/or anti-inflammatory properties, can be potent allergens — as is true for eucalyptus. This is not to say that the various natural ingredients don't have a place in shampoo therapy. On the contrary, we need only look at the example of oatmeal, which has been used to relieve itching and which has no known side-effects (although it's mechanism of action is unknown). But still, oatmeal has in some cases caused an allergic reaction, thereby removing it from the list of hypoallergenic products.

Pet owners and professionals alike should play it safe by doing a little label-research to see if the so-called hypoallergenic products they are using contain any animal proteins, dyes, soaps or perfumes. They should look for all-natural formulations which rely on natural (not man-made) fragrances such as coconut oil. And they should avoid products that use dyes by selecting only those which are clear and transparent. Products that claim to have vegetarian formulations should contain no animal proteins, since animal protein is a major source of antigens in humans and pets who are allergic to animals. Traditionally, animal proteins have been used to provide adhesiveness and better sudsing in shampoo products. That's why a vegetarian formula should be easier to rinse and will not leave behind heavy shampoo buildup.

If the words "cruelty free" appear on the label, it means the product has not been tested on laboratory animals. Even without the animal testing, the Food and Drug Administration (FDA) still considers these formulas as safe to use. Unfortunately, there is not yet an economically feasible way of developing cruelty free tearless shampoos.

Bathing a cat or dog frequently — as often as daily in difficult cases — helps lessen the effects of allergy-causing animal dander or airborne substances such as ragweed. Remember: The pet is literally a dustmop of offending substances to both itself and, potentially, to other pets or people who may be allergic to the same things. That's why it's so important that the shampoo not cause any skin problems. Two highly recommended hypoallergenic shampoos are the DermaPet Conditioning Shampoo and Mycodex HA.

## Oils and Conditioners

Moisturizing agents such as *bath oils, conditioners, emollients* and *humectants* may be applied after bathing and rinsing to soften, lubricate and rehydrate the skin. They can be used on a regular basis for really dry animals. Bath oil is not appropriate for animals with oily skin. Neither are hot oil treatments recommended, for they may be *comedogenic* (causing blackheads). You see, unlike their human counterparts who have simple hair follicles (one hair per pore), dogs and cats have compound hair follicles (multiple hairs growing from each pore). Therefore, a comedogenic product can increase problems by clogging the pores from which multiple hair follicles protrude.

Emollients fill in the spaces between dry skin flakes with oil droplets. They exert their local effect by protecting, softening and increasing the pliability of the skin and serving as vehicles for drugs. Humectants are moisturizing agents that work by trapping transepidermal water. In other words, they prevent water loss. Look for bath oils or conditioners that combine the properties of an emollient and a humectant/moisturizing agent by sealing in moisture and supplying nutrition through fatty acids. Such conditioners can be used daily as moisturizers or topical skin supplements, particularly on animals that swim or live in hot, dry and sunny environments.

Many conditioners and creme rinses now use oatmeal for its anti-itch properties. DermaPet makes both a Conditioner and an Oatmeal Conditioner which contain both humectant and emollient properties. A good conditioner can be used to reduce static electricity and control "flyaway," a condition in which hairs of similar electrical charges repel each other. Some conditioners also may be used in anti-flea dips to assist in insecticide application and to relieve the dryness that often accompanies the use of chemicals — *provided they do not contain a synergist such as sesame seed oil that could turn a normal dip into an overdose.*

## Seborrheic Treatments

Seborrhea is the term used for any skin disease involving dry (sicca) or greasy (oleosa) scaling. The term also encompasses disorders in the formation of keratin, a complex protein unique to the skin, hair follicles and nails. Today, many experts prefer the term "disorders of keratinization." This subject is covered in detail in a separate section of this book. (See Chapter 11.) The epidermis "turns over" every 22 days in the normal dog. Epidermal turnover time in dogs suffering from idiopathic seborrhea (more common among cocker spaniels) may be as little as three to six days. That tremendously rapid turnover creates a defect in the normal protective barrier, which may result in dry or greasy scales, comedones (blackheads), alopecia (hair loss), inflammation, crusts, pyoderma and pruritus (itching). Any of these conditions, in turn, may lead to skin damage. In these cases, it is important to slow the turnover process and treat the secondary problems.

There are many causes of keratinization disorders. Some breeds such as cocker and springer spaniels, Irish setters, basset hounds, West Highland white terriers and Doberman pinschers seem to be predisposed to these primary defects. Secondary causes include ectoparasites (fleas, scabies, *Demodex*, *Cheyletiella*), hormonal disorders (especially hypothyroidism), allergies, dietary defects, environmental factors (dry heat) and skin infections. Generally, a congenital disorder can only be controlled, not cured. But with some secondary disorders, curing the external problem will cure the keratinization disorder. If you eliminate all fleas from the flea-allergic animal, you can then go on to cure the keratinization disorder. However, if the outside cause can be controlled but not completely eliminated, the same will be true for the keratinization disorder. That also would be true for a disorder resulting from an allergic reaction.

The moisturizing effects of water should not be underestimated, particularly when you're dealing with dry and scaling disorders. Contact time of 10 to 15 minutes is enough to hydrate the *stratum corneum*. Be very careful about how much time the animal remains in the water, because dehydration can occur when the contact time is too short; skin maceration (softening) can result when the contact time is too long. In both cases, the protective barrier is damaged. Applying conditioner to the wet coat enhances the moisturizing process.

*Anti-seborrheic* medications usually work as *keratolytic* agents, *keratoplastic* agents or both. A keratolytic agent breaks down the keratin layer. A keratoplastic agent normalizes keratin and epidermal cell formation. Medicated shampoos contain topical agents that have multiple functions, including the control of primary and/or secondary seborrhea. These products often make use of sulfur, salicylic acid, tar, selenium sulfide, benzoyl peroxide and chlorhexidine.

Sulfur is the most common functional, broad-spectrum agent used in medicated shampoos today. It offers keratolytic, keratoplastic, anti-bacterial, anti-parasitic and anti-pruritic functions. There are at least three different types of sulfur: elemental, precipitated and solubilized. This last form is a refined version that allows for a clear, less smelly formulation. With all this, it is still gentle enough that it will not seriously damage the epidermis or hair follicles. However, it should never be used as a replacement for hypoallergenic shampoos when the animal is bathed frequently or cleansed routinely.

Because sulfur is medicinal, it can cause numerous adverse side-effects. Nevertheless, it remains a key component of most overused medicated shampoos, and it does not moisturize. Before turning to such a potentially irritating product, try a moisturizing, soapless shampoo that contains equal parts of solubilized sulfur (two percent) and salicylic acid (two percent), such as DermaPet Seborrheic Shampoo. That's especially true when dealing with cases of dry, scaly seborrhea. Salicylic acid offers keratoplastic, keratolytic, bacteriostatic and mild anti-pruritic functions. When mixed with equal percentages of sulfur, it has a synergistic effect. Although salicylic acid is a compound in many ear-cleansing formulations, it has been identified as ototoxic.

Tar serves as a keratolytic as well as an anti-pruritic, anti-mitotic, anti-inflammatory and degreasing agent. It is overused except perhaps in cases where degreasing is necessary. There are different sources of tar, with pine, juniper and coal tar being the most common. Tar *solutions* are different from *extracted* or *refined* tar because they are diluted. Some of these are filtered to "clear out" the more irritating or aesthetically unpleasant components. In some formulations, the filtering is so extensive that the efficacy of the remaining tar may be questionable. Both shampoo and spray formulations exist at varying concentrations; many shampoos also contain sulfur and/or salicylic acid.

Recently, tar has come under close FDA scrutiny due to its various side-effects, including carcinogenesis. Other potential problems include irritancy, odor, staining and photosensitization. When using a tar formulation, read the label closely. Tar formulations should never be used on cats because felines are incredibly sensitive. Adverse effects of tar may include hair loss or, in extreme cases, death.

Selenium offers anti-bacterial, keratolytic and drying functions. Some experts recommend Selsun Blue to treat *Malassezia* infections. Benzoyl peroxide offers anti-bacterial, keratolytic, anti-pruritic and degreasing functions that may be helpful in treating certain oily skin conditions such as seborrhea oleosa. It also offers follicular flushing, which is important because hair follicles can become infected with bacteria such as *Staphylococcus intermedius*. It is also useful in treating hot spots and pyotraumatic dermatitis.

Hot spots usually are secondary to a predisposing factor such as a flea-bite or an inhalant allergy that causes obsessive scratching, biting, licking or chewing. Hot spots can be treated locally by applying benzoyl peroxide daily to the affected area, allowing it to sit for 10 minutes and then rinsing. Currently, the main benzoyl peroxide-based formulations available for use on pets are DermaPet Benzoyl Peroxide and Benzoyl Peroxide Plus, Mycodex BP (SmithKline Beecham and Norden), Pyoben (Allerderm/Virbac) and Oxidex and Sulfoxidex (DVM). Even among pet-specific products containing only 2.5 to 3 percent benzoyl peroxide, one in 20 can cause side-effects such as irritation. Erythema, irritancy and pain occur more often when highly concentrated human formulations are used. If a side-effect occurs, the area should be cleansed immediately with a hypoallergenic shampoo.

Chlorhexidine, which offers excellent anti-bacterial properties, was a key component in some of the better otic (ear) preparations until it was found to cause deafness and severe ototoxicity and was pulled from the ear medication market by the FDA. On the other hand, chlorhexidine is an excellent choice for the treatment of ringworm or cutaneous yeast infections. It is considered unnecessary for the more common skin infections due to its broad spectrum and inability to flush out hair follicles.

Iodine, used in shampoos for dogs, has anti-bacterial and anti-fungal qualities. I do not recommend using iodine shampoos on cats, however, because felines are incredibly sensitive.

Anti-pruritic formulations vary, and often include many of the ingredients already discussed. Before selecting a product to decrease itching, a pet owner needs to understand what is producing the itching. Eliminating the source of the itch is fundamental. Two of the most common culprits of itching are dryness

| Breed | Grooming Schedule | Brushing | Breed | Grooming Schedule | Brushing |
|---|---|---|---|---|---|
| Afghan | 4-8 weeks | 2x weekly | Keeshonden | 2-3 months | 2x week |
| Airedale | 6-8 weeks | weekly | Kerry Blue | 4-6 weeks | weekly |
| Akita | 3 months | weekly | Labrador Retriever | 3-4 months | weekly |
| Alaskan Malamute | 3 months | weekly | Lhasa Apso | 3-4 weeks | 3x week |
| Basenji | occasional | weekly | Maltese | 3-4 weeks | 3x week, clean eyes |
| Bassett | 2-3 months | face/ears wash weekly | | | |
| | | | Pekingese | 2-3 months | 2x week |
| Beagle | 2-3 months | weekly | Pointers | 2-3 months | weekly |
| Bedlington | 4-6 weeks | weekly | Pomeranian | 2-3 months | prop to thickness |
| Bichon Frise | 4 weeks | weekly | | | |
| Boston Terrier | occasional | weekly | Poodle | 4-6 weeks | varies w. coat, clip & pluck ears |
| Bouvier | 6-8 weeks | weekly | | | |
| Boxer | 2-3 months | weekly | Retrievers | 8-10 weeks | weekly |
| Brittany | 8-10 weeks | weekly | Schnauzer (miniature) | 6-8 weeks | weekly |
| Cairn | occasional | weekly | Scottish Terrier | 6-8 weeks | weekly |
| Chihuahua | occasional | weekly | Shar-Pei | 1-5 weeks | weekly, clean ears |
| Chinese Crested | weekly | apply conditioners regularly | | | |
| | | | Sheepdogs | 6-10 weeks | 3x week |
| Chow | 2-3 months | 2x week | Shih-Tzu | 3-4 weeks | 3x week |
| American Cocker Spaniel | 4-8 weeks | weekly, clean/clip ears | Siberian Husky | 3 months | week |
| | | | Silky Terrier | 3-4 weeks | 3x week |
| Collie (rough) | 6-10 weeks | 3x week | Spaniels | 8-10 weeks | weekly |
| Dachshund | 10-12 weeks | weekly | Springer Spaniel | 8-10 weeks | weekly |
| Dalmatian | 2-3 months | weekly | St. Bernard | 2-3 months | 2x week |
| Doberman | 2-3 months | weekly | Vizslas | 2-3 months | weekly |
| German Shepherd | 2-3 months | weekly | Weimeraners | 2-3 months | weekly |
| Golden Retriever | 8-10 weeks | weekly | West Highland | 3-4 weeks | weekly |
| Greyhounds | 2-3 months | weekly | Yorkshire Terrier | 3-4 weeks | 3x weekly |
| *Frequency always depends upon individual need; seasonally allergic/seborrheic dogs need increased frequency when clinical.* | | | | | |

Table 4.2

and heat. And so, most experts recommend a moisturizing — preferably hypoallergenic — shampoo in *cold* water. If the source is an inhaled allergen carried on a pet's coat, then frequent shampoo sessions are desirable. Oatmeal is considered a natural anti-itch medication.

Anti-parasitic formulations include a broad range of insecticides. I do not recommend flea shampoos, although many will disagree with me. While flea shampoos are less likely to cause toxicity, they also are more likely to be ineffective because they are variably diluted and inconsistently applied. The amount of product used will vary according to the size of the dog, the length of its hair and the bather's preference. And in the end, it all gets rinsed off. The best way to handle parasitic problems is a weekly bath with a hypoallergenic shampoo followed by direct application of an insecticide, preferably in the form of a dip. My personal preference is to use insecticides in the environment rather than on the pet.

## Factors to Consider

When you select a shampoo there are certain factors to consider, including formulation, application, frequency of use and rinsability:

*Formulation.* Select the appropriate formulation from those available after defining the condition to be treated.

*Application.* Apply appropriate products in sequence. First, prepare the coat and skin with a primer shampoo, usually one that is hypoallergenic. Next, apply the selected shampoo and allow the suds to sit on the animal for at least 10 minutes. Use a clock to check the contact time, beginning when the full body is lathered. Contact time will vary according to the product's essential ingredients, its concentration, the condition of the pet's skin and the desired effect. Use of a primer facilitates thorough application of the selected therapeutic product, and decreases the quantity of therapeutic shampoo needed.

*Frequency of use.* Determine how often the shampoo should be applied based on the condition to be treated (or prevented) and the formulation to be used. For example, benzoyl peroxide generally should not be used as a full-body shampoo more often than every three to seven days because it dries out the coat. However, it can be used daily to treat focal lesions such as hot spots, lick granulomas or acne. Formulations containing essential fatty acids, moisturizers and/or conditioners — which actually put more into the coat and skin than they take out — may be used daily to remove topical allergens trapped in the pet's mop-like coat.

*Rinsability.* How well a product rinses from the coat is very important in shampoo therapy, since shampoo build-up can be a primary cause of skin and coat irritation.

# 5

# SKIN INFECTIONS, BACTERIAL AND VIRAL

## Pyoderma and Immunomodulation

*By Dr. Margaret S. Swartout , Knoxville, Tennessee*

B acterial skin infections are a common skin problem in dogs, and less so in cats. They represent the second most common dermatological diagnosis by veterinarians. Called *pyoderma* (pus in the skin), bacterial skin infections can be worrisome, recurring problems that are unsightly and uncomfortable for your pet. Pyodermas may in some circumstances threaten your pet's life if the infection spreads to the internal body parts. But with the help of your veterinarian, and a commitment to proper treatment, pyoderma can usually be resolved. As an informed pet owner, you can be your pet's best friend if pyoderma strikes.

### What You See is What You've Got

Pets affected with pyoderma may have one or many types of skin lesions: red bumps or pimples, bull's-eye target lesions, scabs, flakiness, and skin redness. On a thickly-coated dog, you often feel the bumpiness of lesions before you see them. In many pets, hair loss can be evident in a patchy or "moth-eaten" appearance. It may involve large areas of the body, or it may just look like your pet has a thinning haircoat. In an especially severe deep-skin infection, you might see blood blister-like lesions or even very small crevasse-like openings in the skin which ooze pus or bloody material. With infections involving the feet, cysts sometimes form between the toes or footpads. But there's often more than just what meets the eye! You may also note an excessively oily or dry feel to the skin. A pungent odor may be apparent, caused by microbial growth on the skin and the skin's inflammatory response. For your pet, the most outstanding extravisual symptom is often itchiness.

## The Where and Why

The majority of skin infections do not "just happen;" there is usually a reason why a pet gets a pyoderma. Normally, a pet's immune system should protect it from becoming infected by the bacteria which are around it in the everyday world. There is often an underlying cause which weakens the infected pet's normal defensive abilities against the invading bacteria. In order to help your pet, you will benefit from knowing the underlying cause of the skin infection. For example, parasites such as fleas commonly cause a secondary skin infection. Another problem is mange, a microscopic parasitic infestation that is sometimes difficult to diagnose, but which causes an associated pyoderma.

Endocrine imbalances (most often hypothyroidism, but also Cushing's Syndrome) often leave dogs ripe for a skin infection. Allergic pets are often presented to their veterinarians with skin infections. Patients with seborrhea, a skin condition resulting in excessive flakiness, can also get secondary skin infections. Underlying causes are numerous, and are further listed in Table 5.1. The bottom line for you is to assure that these various predisposing causes of pyoderma are identified and treated in order to optimize the chances of your pet's recovery, and to lessen the likelihood of recurrence.

Remember: If you don't address the underlying cause of pyoderma, it can lead to a failure of even the best treatment program.

## Time for Some Investigation

The principle of underlying cause is very important. Your veterinarian will have the job of identifying the bacterial infection present, and of tracking down the underlying cause. That's why your vet will probably ask you some questions to establish a clinical history. This will be followed by a physical examination, during which the veterinarian will note any lesions, identify any parasites, document hair loss, and look for any other health problems that may make your pet more susceptible to infections of this type. Some testing procedures may help your vet perform this detective work. Your veterinarian may want to make special microscope slide preparations by rubbing or painlessly scraping the skin. Under the microscope, the veterinarian will look for mange mites and

---

## Underlying Causes Of Pyoderma In Pets

- Trauma (bite, scratch wounds)
- Foreign body (buried grass awns or splinters, ingrown hairs)
- Parasites (fleas, mange)
- Hormonal imbalances (hypothyroid, adrenal [Cushing's], sex hormone, growth hormone)
- Allergies (to environmental inhalants, foods, fleas)
- Abnormal skin cell & oil formation (seborrhea, schnauzer comedo)
- Metabolic abnormalities (liver disease, diabetes mellitus)
- Autoimmune diseases (lupus, pemphigus, vasculitis)
- Neoplasia (cancers of many types)
- Nutritional imbalance (poor diet, inability to absorb nutrients)
- Environment (high temperatures and humidity)
- Bacterial hypersensitivity
- Long-term use of corticosteroids
- Sometimes unidentifiable (unfortunately)
- Immune deficiencies (rare)
- Dermatophytes (ringworm)

*Table 5.1*

parasite eggs, and will note the types of cells and microorganisms present. These initial clues about the cause of the skin infection will provide important information about the necessity for further testing and direction of treatment.

If the pyoderma looks serious, or if it is a problem that has reappeared after a previous episode, then bacteriological culturing may be necessary. The purpose of this culture is to identify what bacteria are involved in the skin infection, and to indicate which antibiotics will be effective against these bacteria. We know that the *Staphylococcus intermedius* bacterium is very often the guilty bacterial party, but not all *Staphylococcus* bacteria are alike. It is necessary to identify their particular characteristics and sensitivities to drugs, so that proper treatment can be provided. Moreover, there is no guarantee that the bacterium involved is a *Staphylococcus*; it may be one of a whole variety of other potentially pathogenic bacteria — some quite serious (*Proteus spp*, *Pseudomonas spp*, and *Escherichia coli*). Bacteriological culture of the skin infection is indeed an important clue in finding the microbial agent involved in your pet's skin infection. Other clues are important too. Your veterinarian may propose routine blood counts to evaluate red and white blood cells. Also recommended are other tests that indicate important aspects of your pet's internal health that affect outer health: blood chemistries for evaluating kidney and liver function, and blood sugar measurements to check for diabetes. Moreover, specialized testing may be suggested for thyroid and other hormonal and body functional disorders.

A skin biopsy is a particularly effective method to help determine the depth and severity of the skin infection, and an excellent way to gather information on potential underlying causes of the pyoderma. A minor surgical procedure, a skin biopsy involves taking a very small piece of skin (usually less than half an inch in diameter) while the animal is under local anesthetic. Sometimes a tranquilizer or general anesthesia will be needed to lessen the pet's anxiety. The piece of skin can be examined microscopically by a dermatopathologist, who is a laboratory veterinarian specially trained to examine animal skin biopsies and give interpretation helpful to diagnosis and treatment. The information your veterinarian gathers will indicate not only the type and treatment for the bacteria infecting your pet's skin, but may also point to one or more of the myriad of underlying causes for skin infections.

## Treatment from Inside-Out

One of the most critical treatments for curing pyoderma is the use of antibiotics. The choice of antibiotic is based on several criteria:

- How many times before has pyoderma been a problem for your pet?

- The severity of the pyoderma.

- Laboratory culture identification of bacterial type, and guidelines of antibiotic sensitivity of the bacteria.

Only certain antibiotics are appropriate for treatment of skin infections, either due to their ability to reach the skin after oral administration (through the mouth), or due to their relative effectiveness against bacteria commonly involved in skin infections. Therefore, antibiotics that you may have left over from when your pet had another type of problem might not do the job of eradicating the current pyoderma. It will be up to your veterinarian to choose the appropriate drug. To guarantee success, it is critical that proper antibiotics be given at the appropriate dosage, frequency and length of time. Medications are dosed at various time intervals during the day, depending on important characteristics of appropriate maintenance of blood levels effective for fighting bacteria (see Table 5.2). It is important that the dosage schedule be followed strictly, since under-administration of antibiotics can result in poor efficacy of the drug, and even make the bacteria resistant to that particular antibiotic. For example, if an antibiotic is to be administered three times a day, and is only given twice a day, it may be ineffective (at best) or induce bacterial resistance (at worst). If three-times-a-day antibiotic administration is not possible for you, ask your veterinarian for an antibiotic that is effective when given twice or once a day. Sometimes antibiotics which can be administered less frequently are a bit more costly.

Dosages for antibiotics are calculated based on the pet's weight. Always give the full dose. If the pills are a bad size or shape for your pet, ask if another size or type of drug can be used. Antibiotics should be administered for the proper length of time. Oral antibiotics are carried to the skin by the blood. In comparison to internal organs, the amount of blood that reaches the skin is relatively low. It will take longer for antibiotics to do their work than if the infection were located elsewhere. The surface of the skin will look fine many days before the invisible deeper layers of the skin are cured. It takes at least three weeks of administering an oral antibiotic before the bacterial infection in all layers of the skin is gone. In some very deep or severe infections, it may take even four to 12 weeks or more.

## Antibiotic Administration Frequency

| Prescribed Frequency | When to Give to Your Pet |
|---|---|
| 3 times a day | a.) First thing in the morning<br>b.) Mid-afternoon (or when you get home from work)<br>c.) The third dose at bedtime |
| 2 times a day | a.) First thing in the morning<br>b.) Given about 12 hours later |
| Once a day | Give at the same time each day |

Table 5.2

A good rule of thumb is that antibiotics should be continued a full two weeks after all lesions have disappeared—just to make sure the bacterial infection in the deep areas of the skin has been resolved. Stopping too soon will result in allowing the infection to re-emerge from the deeper layers of the skin. Your veterinarian is the one person most able to determine if the infection is completely cured, so be sure to continue the antibiotics until your re-check visit. Then the veterinarian can let you know whether or not it is safe to stop the medication. Because antibiotics need to be continued for so long in order to cure the pyoderma, it is unlikely that your veterinarian would prescribe injectable antibiotics. There are some uncommon circumstances, involving very serious bacterial infections, in which injectables may be necessary. Your veterinarian should carefully discuss these with you. It is unusual to have side-effects from antibiotics, but it can happen. If for some reason the antibiotic upsets your pet's stomach, or causes some other abnormal symptom, then administering with food or the substitution of another antibiotic may be in order. Ask your veterinarian about these two possibilities.

## Topical Treatments

Treatments applied to the skin can be very important in making your pet feel immediate relief, and in getting rid of the pyoderma. Antibacterial shampoos can effectively reduce skin surface bacterial counts, encouraging skin healing, and making your pet feel better. Common ingredients in these antibacterial shampoos include benzoyl peroxide, chlorhexidine, triclosan, and povidone-iodine. It is important to note that shampoos intended for pets must be used, as those intended for humans are usually too harsh for dogs. In some pets with flaky, oily or dirty skin, a pre-shampoo may be used before the antibacterial shampoo is applies. That guarantees that the antibacterial shampoo comes into close contact with the skin. Your pet's therapeutic shampoo needs may range from treatment every two days to every two weeks. Your veterinarian will tell you the necessary frequency, based on your pet's condition.

Sprays are beneficial to some pets, and will provide temporary relief. Some have soothing ingredients that can be applied directly either through the spray, or by daubing with a wet cotton ball. If there is skin dryness, or if an aggressive shampoo program is needed but likely to promote dryness, a conditioner can also be applied through a spray or by diluting it into the rinse water. Antibacterial creams (containing benzoyl peroxide or mupirocin) may be helpful in some patients with localized pyoderma lesions located in poorly haired areas (such as acne on the chin or lick granulomas).

## Scratch the Itch

What can be done to stop the terrible itching? Relief can take as long as three to five days if the correct antibiotic is used, and if no other disease process which cause itchiness are contributing to the problem. For instance, if your pet is allergic to fleas, and has a secondary pyoderma, it will be necessary to treat the pyoderma *and* institute a thorough flea-control program. Things get more complicated if pets have inhalant allergies, which also cause itchiness. Taking care of the pyoderma will bring some relief, but the pet will still be itchy from the allergies. The animal will need to be tested for allergies, and then put through an allergy therapy program which might involve antihistamines or (as a last resort) corticosteroids. Remember that too many corticosteroids can predispose an animal to pyoderma, an unwanted side-effect. Corticosteroids might inhibit healing, and make it more likely that the skin infection will return.

Remember: The most important thing is to take care of the underlying cause! This may call for antibiotics and antibacterial shampoos for an extended period of time while the veterinarian searches for the primary problem. A cure can only be found when the underlying cause has been identified. All parasites, such as fleas, must be eliminated from both the pet and the animal's environment. Dogs with inhalant allergies should be tested and treated with allergy serum injections, if indicated. Finally, hormonal problems can be solved with medications and other treatments.

# During Recovery: What to Expect

### Hair loss

During recovery, you may see hairs falling out, especially when bathing. Don't worry. These hairs are victims of the skin disease. If the problem has been halted, within an adequate period of time you will probably notice the return of new hair growth. However, some patients have so much skin damage that re-growth of hair is not possible. Only time will tell. If your pet has an underlying cause of the pyoderma which has not been diagnosed (such as a poorly functioning thyroid), hair re-growth usually won't occur until the underlying problem has been addressed.

### Flakiness

You may also notice flakiness during and after the healing stage. This is a normal loss of diseases skin cells as they are replaced by healthy skin cells. Gradually, the flakiness should diminish and stop.

# Is Your Pet Contagious?

Humans can get infections with *Staphylococcus aureus*, a "cousin" of the bacteria which causes pyoderma in pets. However, *Staphylococcus intermedius* which plagues cats and dogs is not considered a threat to humans. It is not really a contagious pathogen to other pets either. The type of *Staphylococcus* that infects our pets is thought to "hang out" on the hair coat of all dogs, and is only allowed to enter the pet's skin to cause a problem when there is an underlying problem which diminishes the skin's ability to keep the bacteria in check.

## Building Immunity

There has been conjecture that several types of drugs would stimulate the immune system, helping the skin fight off infection. As it turns out, few of the patients truly have problems with their immune systems, so trying to stimulate it may be a wasted effort. It is more worthwhile to track down the underlying abnormality which is making your pet more vulnerable to skin infections. However, there are a few selected patients for whom testing has revealed no underlying cause, and who continue to get recurring skin infections which are very itchy. These select patients may be candidates for immune system stimulation. So far, only one type of injectable medication, Staphage Lysate[R], has been found to offer limited effectiveness in boosting the immune system. Treatment can take weeks or months of hypodermic injections.

Be aware that there are cases in which an underlying cause cannot be found or easily rectified (such as ingrown hairs). Moreover, there are certain patients affected with pyodermas that go so deeply into the skin that finding a long-term solution can be quite a challenge. But don't worry, because *most pyodermas can be cured* with appropriate treatment for the bacterial infection, and with attention to identifying and curing the underlying problems. Your efforts in assisting with the detective work, and in the proper administration of treatment, will be critical. As a concerned pet owner, you are the key to your pet's recovery.

# Mycobacteriosis

*By Dr. Alan Mundell, Seattle, Washington*

M ycobacteriosis refers to a group of *rare* diseases caused by bacteria of the genus *Mycobacterium*. All members of this genus have a similar waxy coating, which surrounds the bacterium and imparts a peculiar laboratory staining property called "acid-fast" staining. The coating also makes the organism more resistant to host defense mechanisms and to common antibiotics. Although there are numerous mycobacterial skin diseases, only two are likely to occur among dogs and/or cats in modernized countries.

**Feline leprosy** is caused by *Mycobacterium lepraemurium* (the rat leprosy organism). How the disease is contracted is unknown, but it is believed to be noncontagious to dogs and humans. The disease usually develops in younger roaming cats living in moist coastal areas. There is a long incubation time.

Lesions appear as one or more lumps in or under the skin, especially on the head and legs. If possible, removing the lumps by surgery is preferable, but an experimental treatment using clofazimine may produce a cure if the condition returns. Clofazimine is a new drug which seems to have few side effects.

**Atypical mycobacteriosis** is caused by a group of mycobacteria which differ from other members of the genus because they grow readily on standard bacteria culture media (e.g., blood agar). These organisms usually live harmlessly in soil and water, but in rare instances they may invade traumatized skin. People who work with aquariums seem to be an "at-risk" population. Once the skin is contaminated, any lesions that are produced usually cannot be identified for weeks or months. Skin lesions occur in both dogs and cats; they normally appear as open, non-healing wounds which drain small quantities of fluid. Surgery is recommended to remove infected tissue, but rapid recurrence is common. The pet may respond to long-term antibiotic therapy but is likely to suffer a relapse, often while still on medication. The prognosis for complete cure is guarded, but the outlook for survival is good.

# Viruses as a Cause of Skin Disease

By Dr. Steven A. Melman, Potomac, Maryland

Although frequently cited as a general cause of disease, viruses are apparently rare in dogs and cats. Nevertheless, in some cases — Feline Immunodeficiency Virus (FIV) and Feline Leukemia Virus (FeLv) — a diagnosis may be devastating to an otherwise uninformed owner. The following is a brief overview of viral diseases which affect the skin.

## Feline Leukemia Virus (FeLv)

FeLv is highly prevalent and is well known for its immunosuppressive effects in cats. Although studies have not shown any direct relationship, chronic and recurrent skin infections (pyodermas, abscesses and cellulitis) have been observed. These infections represent an ineffective immune response to fight off a normal bacterial infection. In cats, *Pasteurella multocida* may cause abscesses (pockets of infection filled with pus in the skin, which are walled off) and cellulitis (a deep and severe infection which gets in between the tissues—even in healthy animals). FeLV infected cats are less likely to have an effective immune response, and therefore more likely to have these sorts of infections.

Paronychia (an infection around the nail), poor wound healing, seborrhea and pruritus (itchiness) also may occur. Multiple cutaneous horns have been found on the footpads of cats with FeLV.

*FeLv is believed to rank second (after trauma) among the most common causes of death of cats in the United States.* It is a retrovirus which can be diagnosed by ELISA or IFA (immunofluorescence). ELISA is most commonly done in veterinary offices. The IFA is less likely to have a false positive result, but is also more likely to be false negative, since a positive result requires an advanced and serious state of infection. Cats which have had negative ELISA tests are commonly vaccinated against FeLv.

## Feline Immunodeficiency Virus (FIV)

FIV was first discovered in California in 1986 in a cattery. Its incidence can be as high as 14 percent among ill cats and as low as 1.4 percent among the general population in North America. Often, cats afflicted with FeLv also have FIV. Although FIV appears to be related to Simian and Human Immunodeficiency viruses, it is probably more like other viruses. Fortunately for man, it is specific to one species only (in this case, cats), as is true with other lentiviruses. However, FIV is progressive and lifelong. It is found in saliva, blood, cerebrospinal fluid and does not live well in the environment off the animal. *Biting is the only proven method of transmission.*

Due to their roaming nature, males are twice as likely as females to become infected. Cats are usually five years young or more. No studies have shown that the virus is transmitted to kittens via the uterus or by breast feeding. Fever, lymph node enlargement and a low white blood cell count (mainly, T cells are depleted) are the common early signs. The most common clinical signs are diseases of the gums: chronic gingivitis, stomatitis and periodontitis. Chronic diseases and opportunistic infections are the hallmarks of this syndrome. *Demodex* mites, or demodectic mange (See Chapter 7), may be found on cats infected with FIV. Diagnoses by ELISA tests, which are most commonly used by veterinary practices and some labs, are marred with 20 to 30 percent false positives. This is due to nonspecific cross-reacting antibodies. Western Blot analysis is much more specific. Kittens 10 weeks of age and under will have antibodies from infected mothers, which disappear.

## Feline Pox Virus

This virus is believed to be similar to the one which causes cowpox—an orthopox of the same class that causes smallpox. Lesions consists of ulcers, papules, pustules and plaques. *Similar signs have been reported in humans exposed to infected cats.* Systemic illness may or may not occur. The diagnosis is made by biopsy of the infected tissue and microscopic exam. For more specific diagnosis, electron microscopy is needed. To be identified, the virus must be isolated (preferably) from the scab.

## Transmissible Venereal Tumor

Also known as contagious venereal tumor, transmissible venereal tumor is an uncommon benign tumor of dogs which sometimes can be malignant. It is most often transmitted by sexual contact, but also by licking, biting and scratching. The tumor is more common in temperate climes and in large urban areas where roaming animals may be more prevalent. The tumor cells are characterized by an unusual number of chromosomes (59) as opposed to the normal number in dogs (78). *Experts suspect a virus may be the cause, but this has not been confirmed.* Interestingly, when a modified live parvovirus vaccine was inoculated at the same time as this presumed virus, no growth of tumor was seen.

Neoplasms occur commonly on the penis and vagina, where they may appear as giant cauliflower-like masses which may be ulcerated and bleeding. Lesions may also appear on the face, limbs and other areas of the skin. The tumor's characteristic behavior remains unknown and variable, with occasional regression. Although laboratory-infected dogs appear to regress close to 90 percent of the time, the tumor's unusual behavior in naturally occurring infections leads most experts to recommend vigorous therapy, ranging from surgery to radiation and/or chemotherapy. The tumor is not contagious to man.

## Cutaneous Papillomas

Cutaneous Papillomas are common in dogs and rare in cats. They are benign tumors arising from skin cells. There are various causes, of which two variants are caused by a DNA papovavirus. They are *canine viral papillomatosis* and *cutaneous inverted papillomas.*

- •Canine viral papillomatosis is a contagious disease which only affects young dogs. Multiple lesions are the rule. They vary in size from papules to large, narrow-based, cauliflower-like masses. The lesions mainly affect the head and mucous membranes. They should not be confused with the multiple tiny masses that commonly occur in older male dogs (mainly cockers and Kerry blue terriers) and cats.

- •Cutaneous inverted papillomas occur on the ventrum of dogs from eight months to three years of age. They are raised and firm, and contain a central pore which opens to the skin.

Papillomas may transform into *squamous cell carcinomas*. (See Chapter 18) Clinical management usually involved surgery except in the case of *canine viral papillomatosis*, which usually regresses within three months. Other viruses include *canine distemper* (paramyxovirus) which can cause a thickened nose or foot pad, known as *hardpad disease*. Some dogs were found to be infected with *Orf* (a paravaccinia) virus. This causes a syndrome known as contagious viral pustular dermatitis, with ulcers and crusts occurring mainly around the head. Diagnosis is the same as for pox virus. This virus is also contagious to humans.

Feline *herpes* virus has been associated with oral and skin ulcerations in cats. The ulcerations appear on all areas of skin, including footpads. Feline *calici* virus is known as *"paw and mouth"* disease. Lesions affect the foot, which can be swollen, and the mouth, where blisters can be found on the tongue, lips and palate.

# 6

# MYCOLOGY

## Fungal Diseases that Affect the Skin

*By Dr. Steven A. Melman, Potomac, Maryland*

Of the thousands of different fungal species, only a handful are able to cause disease in animals. Most fungi are soil organisms or plant pathogens. Nevertheless, that "handful" of animal-loving fungi numbers approximately 300 species. Based on clinical reports, one of the most common animal-attacking fungi in veterinary medicine is the mysterious "grass fungus." The grass fungus is somewhat like a joke in which a person brags he can speak any language in the world except Greek. When asked to say something in Tibetan, the braggart then replies, "Nope, that one's Greek to me!" In the same vein, whenever many clinicians are unable or unwilling to make a firm diagnosis, they will shrug off further investigation by labeling the rogue a "grass fungus." Invariably, more detailed examination would probably reveal that the true cause of all the patient's problems is a contact allergy, an inhalant allergy or a myriad of other hypersensitivities. Many cases would even turn out to be simple antibiotic-responsive pyodermas. Grass fungus is an easy diagnosis to fall back on. After all, making a final and accurate diagnosis is not easy, given the presence of multiple symptoms involved in fungal diseases. This is further complicated by the constantly changing science of nomenclature, which makes it nearly impossible for veterinarians to keep up with the latest "shifts" and "re-categorizations."

For the purpose of easy discussion, this chapter will include the latest names of the various fungi species that affect our dogs and cats. We will ignore most synonyms and previous scientific names. Some lists will be provided, with a bibliography that you are encouraged to use. Those fungal diseases discussed in this chapter include mycetoma, pseudomycetoma, and subcutaneous mycoses such as Blastomycosis, Histoplasmosis, Cryptococcosis and Coccidioidomycosis, as well as Sporotrichosis.

## Some Definitions

**Mycosis**: This is a disease caused by a fungus.

**Dermatomycoses**: These are fungal diseases (-mycoses) that affect the skin (dermato-). They tend to be differentiated from the dermatophytoses (ringworm) which only grow in keratinizing epithelium (the top layer of skin) and which cannot proliferate or survive in living, growing tissue (see page 78, Ringworm).

**Fungi**: There are five kingdoms of organisms: Fungi; Animalia (animals), Protista (protozoa), Monera (algae) and Plantae (plants). Fungi are characterized by their nucleus, and lack of chlorophyll in their cell walls. Fungi may grow as a yeast (single cell) or mold (multicellular), and in many cases both.

**Dimorphic Fungi**: Those fungi which grow as both yeast and mold are classified as dimorphic. Those that grow in warm tissue are called yeasts, while those growing in the natural environment are molds.

**Cell-Wall Components**: The components of the fungal cell wall include chitin, chitosan, glucan and mannan. These components help differentiate fungi from algae.

**Fungi Classes**: There are five classes of fungi — Ascomycota; Basidiomycota; Chytridomycota; Deuteromycota or Fungi Imperfecti; and Zygomycota. The Fungi Imperfecti and Ascomycota are the primary pathogens in animals.

**Classification**: Fungi are further defined by their methods of sexual reproduction (either *sexual* or *asexual*), the appearance of the units in terms of nuclei, types of growth, color, cell divisions and other biochemical and immunological characteristics.

**Diagnosis Confirmation**: Fungi can usually be seen in histopathologic specimens obtained via biopsy. Nevertheless, the only way to confirm a diagnosis of fungal disease is to culture, grow and identify the fungal organism. Proper specimen collection by a trained veterinarian is mandatory. Note — Ringworm and *Malassezia* are featured in other sections of this book. For more information on Ringworm and *Malassezia*, turn to pages 78 and 83, respectively.

**Subcutaneous Mycoses**: Nomenclature can be confusing, and what is printed here may easily become "reclassified" by the experts in taxonomy. Nevertheless, according to the leading textbook in the field of veterinary dermatology (Muller, Kirk and Scott's *Small Animal Dermatology*), the "cutaneous mycoses and their infective agents" include:

- Eumycotic mycetoma (*Pseudoallescheria boydii, Curvelaria geniculata*): tissue grains, draining fistulae and swelling.

- Prototheca (*Prototheca wickerhamii*): Supposedly this organism was previously described as from Monera (blue-green algae). Although rare, they are considered achloric variants of green algae.

- Pithyosis (*Pythium sp.*): Referred to as the correct name for what was once known as belonging to the protozoans.

- Rhinosporidosis

- Sporotrichosis (*Sporotrix schenkii*): This may also cause systemic disease.

- Zygomycota

**Mycetoma**: These are swollen, draining lesions in the subcutaneous tissue which contain granules or tissue "grains." They are rare — usually caused by a traumatic penetrating wound, localized to one area of the body (typically a limb or the abdomen). They may also be a member of the actinomycetes. If not caused by fungi or actinomycetes, they result from a dermatophyte or nonactinomycete bacteria — thereby being termed *pseudomycetoma*.

Both mycetoma and pseudomycetoma may be confused with normal abscesses (which should respond to drainage and antibiotics) and foreign bodies (such as foxtails, awns or thorns). Atypical mycobacteria and feline leprosy should also be included in the differential diagnosis. Histopathology obtained by a biopsy usually tells the story. Treatment can be difficult, depending on the organism. Early lesions usually respond quite well to surgical removal. More advanced cases may require amputation or deep surgical removal and curettage with antifungal drugs (which are usually ineffective).

## Systemic Mycoses

These organisms are grouped as primary (P) and secondary (S). The primary fungi can invade animal tissues and cause infection, while the secondary organisms usually cause infections only in hosts already suffering from a compromised immune system.

| Organism | P/S | Habitat |
|----------|-----|---------|
| Blastomyces dermatitidis | P | Humis, rich soils such as those along the Mississippi and Ohio rivers. |
| Histoplasma capsulatum | P | Soil contaminated by bat, chicken and bird feces. |
| Coccidioides immitis | P | Semi-arid soil, as in the deserts of the Southwest. |
| Cryptococcus neoformans | S | Pigeon droppings and contaminated soil. |

Table 6.1

**Systemic Mycoses:** These are fungal infections of internal organs that may spread to the skin. Not usually pathogenic, they normally exist in soil and vegetation. These fungi are normally found in localized, endemic areas where they come in contact with many animals. However, only a few animals become ill because of these systemic mycoses. Some of these organisms — known as secondary pathogens — may be more likely to cause symptoms of infection in animals that are in some way "compromised" immunologically. The use of immunosuppressive agents such as prednisone, for example, can lead to such a problem. The mycoses may also cause skin problems in patients undergoing chemotherapy, as well as those suffering from diseases such as feline leukemia, feline immunodeficiency virus, canine distemper, hypervitaminosis A, diabetes mellitus, lymphosarcoma and leukemia. While these organisms are not considered contagious, the fungal colonies they produce in culture can cause a disease in humans.

**Blastomycosis:** This illness is caused by the *Blastomyces* fungi. These fungal organisms are dimorphic, meaning they can survive in tissue as yeasts, and outside (depending on temperature) as molds. They are quite common along the Ohio and Mississippi river basins. They can cause a full-body (systemic) infection that will, in 40 percent of all cases, affect the skin. The dog is the most likely victim, with reported cases of feline infections quite rare. Infection (both through external invasion and internal spread) typically affects the head, legs, scrotum and chest. Localized-to-regional lymph node enlargement is often dramatic. Skin lesions are usually chronic bumps (papules) that may vary in size and become ulcerated (losing their outer layer of skin). They may contain draining tracts (fistulae) that release a mixed pus-and-serous discharge. Diagnosis is made by identifying the organism through either the tissue or its discharge. The prognosis is guarded. Vigorous treatment involving antifungal drugs, such as amphotericin, requires hospitalization. Although not believed to be highly contagious to humans, people have been infected from culture of the organism and from a dog bite.

**Histoplasmosis:** Caused by a dimorphic fungus that thrives in soil contaminated with bird, bat and chicken droppings (with a high incidence in river valleys from the Midwest and Southern states), this ailment rarely affects the skin. However, when it does, the result is nodules. Diagnosis is most often made by biopsy, and treatment is similar to that for blastomycosis.

**Coccidioidomycosis:** Seen mainly in the desert regions of the United States, this ailment is also known as Valley Fever. It can strike some animals with symptoms, while remaining asymptomatic in others. Be very careful when handling cultures, since they form giant endospores which are highly contagious to both humans and animals. Consequently, materials taken for culture should be placed on a special growth media and sent to a laboratory equipped to handle such hazardous materials. The skin is usually not involved. The lesions may appear as abscesses, with fistulas or nodules known as granulomas. Treatment is the same as for blastomyces.

**Cryptococcosis:** This is a fairly common yeast believed to live in soil contaminated by pigeon droppings, and is more often found in warmer climates. It is a saprophyte, meaning it thrives on dead or decaying matter. However, it is an opportunist — a secondary infector that may cause infection in immunocompromised animals. Cryptococcosis is the most commonly diagnosed systemic mycosis of cats, although it is less frequent in dogs. Experts speculate that this is because cats more commonly frequent places where there may be pigeon droppings. Clinical signs usually involve lesions on the head (these can be solitary, or they can cover the entire body), tiny papules or nodules which can ooze and ulcerate (although they may become crusted over, and appear to be healing). Or else they can appear as abscesses or fluid-filled nodules. Lymph nodes may become enlarged.

Diagnosis can be made by cytology of the lesion exudate, or by biopsy tissue (which may require a unique type of stain used by trained pathologists). A blood test (the latex agglutination test) for cryptococcal antigens can be useful in supporting the diagnosis and following the progress of the disease and/or treatment. Because the prognosis is guarded, treatment can be difficult. Recently, the use of ketaconazole and iatroconazole has shown some promise, especially with the aid of surgical excision whenever possible.

# Dermatophytosis (Ringworm)

*By Dr. Linda Medleau, Athens, Georgia*

Ringworm is a fungal infection of the skin, hair or nails. In most instances of canine and feline ringworm, the cause can be traced directly to *Microsporum gypseum*, *Microsporum canis*, or *Trichophyton mentagrophytes*. Of the three, only *M. gypseum* makes its home in the soil. *M. canis* and *T. mentagrophytes*, meanwhile, are specialized parasites that live on the skin of animals. In fact, *M. canis* is so well adapted to cats that it may live on their hair and skin without causing any sign of disease. Pets can become infected with *M. gypseum* when they come in contact with contaminated soil. But these infections occur sporadically, and are not easily passed between animals — unlike infections from *M. canis*, which can spread quite easily among animals in close contact with each other. *M. canis* infections may also be spread indirectly through contact with contaminated objects, such as brushes or shared furniture. That's why the infection may spread rapidly in a litter of puppies confined in a small, unsanitary area.

The sudden development of ringworm in a litter of kittens or any other recently acquired animal is often the first clue that a resident adult cat has a "subclinical" infection. The adult feline may not be showing signs of ringworm, but the fungi are there, ready to attack the more susceptible younger generation. Exposure to ringworm does not always result in infection, thanks in part to "washing away" of the fungal spores, unsuccessful competition with already established normal skin flora, and the animal's immunologic resistance. When the ringworm organism is able to penetrate the skin or invade hair follicles, overcoming the pet's immune defense mechanisms, an infection will follow.

# Recognizing Ringworm

There are many varied clinical signs to help owners recognize a ringworm infection. Quite often, pet owners may not know their cats are infected with *M. canis* until the ringworm has spread to humans in the household. The owners will then examine the family cat more carefully, and discover areas of partial hair loss, scaling or broken-off hairs. Ringworm is not normally an itchy disease, but there are cases where it has been mildly-to-strongly itchy.

In cats, the typical sign of ringworm is a crusty, circular area of hair loss. Cats may appear to have only one or two areas of infection, but hairs that appear normal elsewhere on the body are usually also infected. On kittens, ringworm usually makes its first appearance as circular areas of hair loss on the face, ears or front legs. On adult cats, ringworm may first show itself as a small area of hair loss, several patchy areas of hair loss, or diffuse hair loss across the entire body. Affected skin may also be scaly, crusty and reddened.

In dogs, the ringworm lesions show a great deal of variation. Clinical signs may include papules, hair loss, skin redness, scales and crusts. They may range from barely visible scaly patches of partial hair loss with little evidence of inflammation, to raised, red nodules called *kerions*. The amount of lesions may also vary, from one to many. Sometimes the entire body may be affected. Ringworm rarely causes infection of the nails, but when it does the nails become dry, brittle and deformed.

# Diagnose, Then Treat

Because ringworm is not too common, the veterinarian should make a positive diagnosis before beginning any treatment program. To this end, the veterinarian can use an ultraviolet light exam, skin scrapings of scales and hairs, skin biopsies, and fungal cultures. An ultraviolet light — called the Wood's light — is used for a quick screening. The animal is placed in a darkened room, and its haircoat examined under the light. Hairs invaded by some strains of *M. canis* will glow (fluoresce) a yellow-green color. But this isn't an all-conclusive method of diagnosis, since not all strains of *M. canis* fluoresce, while *M. gypseum* and *T. mentagrophytes* never fluoresce. On top of that, the use of certain topical medications such as iodine may prevent fluorescence.

Therefore, lack of fluorescence does not rule out ringworm. Then again, there are also some topical ointments and solutions which may cause fluorescence, regardless of the presence of *M. canis*. After all this, why bother with ultraviolet light? Well, the Wood's light is best used as an aid in choosing which hairs to scrape for a microscopic exam or fungal culture. Examining skin scrapings and hairs from lesions may be more helpful in making a diagnosis. Veterinarians will study the hairs and scales under a microscope, looking for fungal spores. Unfortunately, fungal spores are hard to see, and false negative results are common.

The most reliable method for diagnosing ringworm is the fungal culture. Veterinarians can either pluck hairs and scales from skin lesions, or they can use the "toothbrush technique." The toothbrush technique is especially useful in identifying infected cats that have no lesions. It involves combing the animal's entire body. This combing should be aggressive enough so that the brush comes away with a collection of hairs, which are then cultured.

Once the diagnosis of ringworm is unquestionably positive, it is time to begin treatment. The treatment method depends in part on a number of variables, including the nature of the infection and the animal's environment:

### Localized Ringworm

When the animal has only a few areas of infection on the body, there is a possibility that the problem will be self-limiting. Therefore, the animal may get better on its own. Then again, the infection may spread to other areas on the body, or to other animals and people. When localized ringworm is diagnosed, the lesion should be clipped.

A topical antifungal product is applied once or twice a day to the lesions and the hairs immediately surrounding it to prevent the spread of infection. Treatment is continued one week past the apparent clinical cure. Antifungal products that may be used in treating localized lesions include thiabendazole solution, providone-iodine ointment, chlorhexidine ointment, miconazole cream or solution, haloprogin cream or solution, econazole cream, and clotrimazole cream. There are also several topical products that are effective in human ringworm, but have not been tested on dogs or cats. These products include ketoconazole cream, sulconazole nitrate cream and solution, oxiconazole nitrate cream, and naftifine hydrochloride cream. Animals that do not improve with localized topical treatment should be treated for generalized ringworm infection.

### Generalized Ringworm

When the infection has spread to multiple areas on the body, treatment is usually necessary. While cats may appear to have only localized lesions, they can possibly have infected hairs elsewhere on the body. Therefore, culturing the entire haircoat using the toothbrush technique should be done to rule out the possibility of generalized ringworm. If it is determined that animals with medium or long haircoats have generalized ringworm, the hair should be clipped with a No. 10 blade. The entire body should then be treated with a topical antifungal solution (dip) once or twice a week until fungal cultures are negative, or two weeks past clinical cure. Treatment may demand a minimum of four weeks.

Antifungal products for the topical treatment of generalized fungal lesions include lime sulfur solution (Lymdip), chlorhexidine solution (Nolvasan) and povidone-iodine solution (Betadine). One warning: Povidone-iodine may be especially irritating to feline skin. Jewelry should be removed and protective clothing, including rubber gloves, should be worn by the person doing the treatment. The solution should be applied to the animal's body with a sponge until the haircoat and skin are completely saturated. The entire body is treated, including the face, but contact with the eyes should be avoided. The solution is not rinsed off, but is allowed to air dry on the animal.

If topical treatment alone is not enough, the veterinarian may decide it is time to add oral antifungal drugs to the regimen. For oral treatment, griseofulvin is the drug of choice because it has been approved for use in both cats and dogs. Griseofulvin is poorly absorbed unless given with a high-fat meal. It must also be administered daily to be effective. Griseofulvin (Fulvicin-U/F) may be prescribed at a dosage of 25 mg per pound once a day, or half that amount twice daily. If no improvement is seen after two weeks of treatment with griseofulvin, the dosage should be doubled. Griseofulvin is teratogenic, which means it can cause fetal mutations and deformed offspring. It should therefore not be given to pregnant animals. Nausea, vomiting or diarrhea occasionally develop, and can be alleviated by administering the griseofulvin in two or three divided daily doses.

Idiosyncratic (unpredictable) reactions in cats have also been reported, including anemia, low white blood cell count, low platelet count, jaundice, fever, depression, muscle weakness and itching. To monitor cats for adverse reactions, the veterinarian should take counts of both red and white blood cells, as well as platelets, every other week during treatment. If signs of griseofulvin side-effects develop, the drug should be stopped. With the possible exception of muscle weakness, side-effect signs should resolve after griseofulvin treatment is ended.

Ketoconazole (Nizoral) and itraconazole (Sporanox) are also effective in treating ringworm, but neither drug is approved for animal use. The administration of ketoconazole or itraconazole—recommended dosages of 5 to 10 mg per pound once a day or half that amount twice daily — is usually effective. Giving the medicine with food will enhance its absorption. Treatment must continue until fungal cultures are negative, or for two weeks beyond clinical cure. Effective treatment usually demands at least four weeks.

Side-effects of ketoconazole and itraconazole included decreased appetite, vomiting, diarrhea, weight loss, elevated liver enzyme levels, jaundice and death. Veterinarians should monitor liver enzyme levels every two to four weeks during treatment, because an increase in liver enzyme levels may occur long before any recognizable clinical signs arise. Reversible lightening of the haircoat has also been described in dogs receiving ketoconazole treatment. And because mummified fetuses and stillbirths have been documented in bitches treated with ketoconazole, the medicine should not be used with pregnant animals.

The effects of itraconazole on pregnant animals is as yet unknown. If any side-effects are suspected, treatment should be stopped and the animal's liver enzyme levels must be measured. Animals may need supportive care, such as fluid therapy, until they recover. Treatment can be reinstituted at a lower dosage, or given every other day — perhaps both — after the liver enzyme levels normalize and the animal's normal appetite returns. This will usually take a couple of weeks at the most. Dividing the total daily dosage into two or three doses may help prevent appetite loss and vomiting. Itraconazole is more expensive than ketoconazole, but it has fewer side-effects — especially in cats. Because only griseofulvin is approved for use in both dogs and cats, it should be the initial choice. However, ketoconazole or itraconazole treatment can be considered as alternatives in case the animal develops a resistance or intolerance to griseofulvin.

### Multiple-pet Environments

When more than one dog or cat is involved, the infected animals need to be separated from the non-infected ones. Things become tricky in a multiple-cat or cattery situation, because subclinically infected cats must be identified. Hairs from all cats must be collected for fungal culturing using the toothbrush method. But a separate brush and culture must be used for each cat. Culture-positive animals must be clipped and separated from their culture-negative companions.

If a large number of animals are infected, the least expensive treatment is with topical antifungal dips once or twice weekly — including those pets that culture-tested negative. Any dog with ringworm and all cats (including previously culture-negative cats) are re-cultured for ringworm every two to four weeks. To prevent re-infections, treatment is normally continued for at least a month after all animals are culture-negative. At the start of the treatment regimen, the pet owner should be aware that topical therapy alone may not work, and that oral antifungal therapy may need to be added at a later date.

If topical therapy alone is proving ineffective, a more aggressive approach is called for. All infected animals should be clipped, treated topically, and treated orally with griseofulvin. Exposed, non-infected animals can be treated prophylactically with griseofulvin — 25 mg per pound, daily for 10 to 14 days. In cattery situations, all cats should be treated. Because griseofulvin is contra-indicated in pregnant animals, females cannot be bred during treatment. Also, the cats should not be shown or loaned for breeding purposes, and new animals should not be introduced into the colony during the treatment period. Treatment should continue until lesions are gone, and fungal cultures are negative in all animals. If there are several animals to take care of, the treatment program can become quite expensive.

## Preventative Measures

Infected hairs must be removed from the environment so that re-infection does not occur. Carpets and furniture should be vacuumed once or twice a week. In cattery and kennel situations, the heating ducts, ceiling, ventilation ducts, and transportation vehicles should be vacuumed. Floors, countertops, windowsills, litter boxes and any other hard surfaces that the animals have come in contact with should be disinfected once or twice weekly with a bleach solution diluted 1:10 in water. Cages and carriers should be cleaned each day with chlorhexidine solution diluted 1:4 in water. Grooming tools and toys should also be disinfected or destroyed.

To prevent a subclinically infected cat from starting a ringworm outbreak, owners should isolate and get fungal cultures from all newly acquired pets, cats that have been at shows, and cats that have been loaned to other catteries. Newly acquired puppies with skin lesions should also be isolated until it is determined they do not have ringworm. Suspect animals should be prophylactically treated with topical antifungal shampoos or dips every five days, depending on culture results.

Because ringworm is a zoonotic (contagious to humans) disease, strict hygiene is required when treating infected animals. Infected pets should have limited contact with people, especially young children and the elderly. Owners should wear gloves whenever handling infected pets, and wash their hands afterwards. People who develop ringworm should contact their physicians for appropriate treatment.

# Cutaneous Malassezia (yeast)

*By Dr. Michael Shipstone, Queensland, Australia*

Malassezia is the name given to a particular yeast organism that lives on the skin of your pet. It is a perfectly normal part of the group of organisms that live on animal skin, and is not the result of negligence on the part of the pet owner. Unfortunately, some pets react to the yeast in an abnormal way — scratching or chewing themselves. The body may also try to rid itself of the yeast by producing extra layers of skin, which are then shed off. The irritation of this may lead the skin to increase the production of grease and oil. Some or all of these symptoms may be present in your pet. Malassezia is a common disease, although it is only quite recently that the role of this yeast in the clinical picture has been recognized. Your veterinarian can perform a number of different tests to determine whether or not your pet's skin is under siege by the *Malassezia* yeast:

### Cytology

The veterinarian will use either a scalpel blade or sticky tape to transfer some of the surface layers of skin to a glass microscope slide, which will then be stained using special dyes (Diff-Quik) to show the characteristically peanut-shaped yeast organisms. Quite often, the yeast is also accompanied by an overgrowth of *Staphylococcus*, a normal skin bacteria.

### Biopsy

Your veterinarian may need to take a small round punch of skin, which is sent to a laboratory for processing. The *Malassezia* sometimes may be seen on the biopsy, but even if it is not, it causes a characteristic change to the pathology of the skin which can be seen and recognized by the pathologist. When taking a biopsy of the skin, the veterinarian will leave the scale layer intact. This means the only pre-biopsy preparation necessary is a hair-trimming. No skin disinfectants should be used.

### Therapy Response

The way your pet responds to a specific therapy can often determine whether or not it has a disease. Malassezial dermatitis may be *secondary* to some other conditions (such as allergy), but the clinical signs of the dermatitis mask the primary cause. Removal of the secondary seborrhea dermatitis will make it

---

## *Clinical Signs of Malassezia Overgrowth*

*Pets afflicted with an irritating overgrowth of Malassezia yeast will display the following symptoms:*

| | |
|---|---|
| • *Generalized itchiness* | • *Generalized redness* |
| • *Face rubbing* | • *Formation of scale and dandruff* |
| • *Foot chewing* | • *Thickening of the skin* |
| • *Irritation of the lower back and bottom of the tail* | • *Loss of hair, baldness in some cases* |
| | • *Eye irritation* |

Table 6.2

easier for the veterinarian to recognize and treat the primary or main condition that is causing the dog to scratch, chew or flake.

The yeast organism is commonly found in the ears, around the face, between the toes, around the vulva and under the tail. But it may be found all over the body (particularly in West Highland terriers). Affected animals are "greasy," and have a characteristic rancid, offensive odor caused by the action of yeast and bacteria. The method of treatment chosen by the veterinarian depends in large part on the severity of the clinical signs, and on how long the yeast has been growing on the animal.

### Mild Cases

When the animal hasn't been affected for long, or when the condition is secondary to some other problem, treatment should be relatively simple. The veterinarian may recommend a topical medication, such as Mycodex, Benzoyl Peroxide or DermaPet Benzoyl Peroxide Plus. These may be applied twice a week until the condition is under control, when the treatment can be cut back to once a week or as necessary.

### Chronic Cases

More intensive therapy may be necessary when the condition has been going on for a long time, as evidenced by skin thickening, hair loss, increased scale formation, increased sebum production, and a strong odor. At this stage, the animal may be given tablets that will kill both the yeast and bacteria. A typical prescription may include Nizoral and Clavamox, to be given between four and six weeks, perhaps. This long course of therapy is necessary to kill all organisms, and to allow the skin a chance to return to normal (regrow) without having to fight the organisms. If the therapy is not carried to its full length, the yeast and accompanying bacterial growths will take over again once the antibiotics have worn off.

While your pet is taking its tablets, it will also need the regular baths in the medications named above. These treatments are designed to remove the scale and grease from the coat, and reduce the number of organisms growing on the skin. This dual treatment speeds up the recovery, quickly bringing the condition under control until it is fully eradicated.

# One Final Word of Advice

What is important for all pet owners to understand is that these yeast organisms are a normal part of the populations of bugs that live on animal skin.

The only problem is that some individual pets are not able to handle even normal numbers of organisms without some problems, such as scratching. So even if the veterinarian is successful in treating your pet and getting the symptoms under control, it does not mean the pet will never have the same problem again. Sadly, some animals require constant treatments for life (including weekly medicated baths) to be able to live a normal existence, while other pets need only periodic treatments. Then, too, there are the lucky animals that need just one course of therapy to reach a normal life, and there they stay for the rest of their days.

# Sporotrichosis

*By Dr. Steven A. Melman, Potomac, Maryland*

Of the many skin diseases that can plague dogs, few are communicable to humans. Sporotrichosis is one exception. Caused by the fungal organism *Sporothrix schenkii*, the disease is considered a public health hazard because of its ability to spread rapidly through the human community. In fact, in 1989 a number of states were hit with an outbreak of Sporotrichosis that was spread by the Sphagnum moss used to pack seedlings in Wisconsin. The moss provided a good home for *S. schenkii*, which can exist as either a yeast in skin or as a mold (mycelium) on decaying organic matter — such as moss or soil. The disease is much more common in cats than dogs. Sadly for cats, the organism thrives in feline tissue and exudates, such as feces. The public health ramifications of this are obvious, given the growing popularity of cats as pets.

Increasingly, the cat is now considered an important source of human infection. That's why people handling infected cats need to wear disposable gloves, and wash their forearms and hands with a disinfectant such as chlorhexadine or betadine. Sporotrichosis is most commonly seen in hunting dogs and cats, usually associated with a puncture wound. This may account for the predisposition of the disease in male cats that roam the neighborhood.

## The Disease in Dogs

There are three major forms of the disease as it manifests itself in canines. *The disseminated form* of sporotrichosis is rare. It may show up as a nodule which can ulcerate and develop draining tracts. The veterinarian should become suspicious when an ailing dog does not respond to a typical course of antibiotics. *The cutaneous form* usually appears as multiple nodules on the head or trunk that may ulcerate, develop draining tracts and crust over. The infection ascends proximally (toward the head) and may lead to other similar lesions. *The cutaneo-lymphatic form* is usually quite similar to the cutaneous form, but with lymph node involvement (typically manifested as swelling of an extremity).

## The Disease in Cats

The sporotrichosis disease is especially ugly and vicious in cats, behaving somewhat differently than it does with canines. In cats, the organism usually disseminates rapidly throughout the organ systems. It is profuse as it exudes from draining tracts, feces and tissues. Lesions usually occur in areas most likely to have abscesses resulting from fight wounds. Normally cats take a beating on the head, tail base, face and the farthest points (the distal aspects) of the limbs. Most feline-infected sporotrichosis patients find their way to the veterinary clinic with infected battle wounds that will not heal. Such cases usually form multiple nodules which ulcerate, drain a serous exudate, and may crust over. The cat's normal grooming behavior helps spread the disease organism and lesions all over the body.

Even though the presence of lymph node involvement is easily seen on a living cat's physical examination, autopsies will give evidence of cording (the presence of organisms filling up the lymphatic vessels and cells as they drain through the system). And if the organisms are found in many other organ systems, as well as the feces, you can bet that they've already disseminated themselves throughout the body. Signs of systemic infection in both cats and dogs include lethargy, anorexia (loss of appetite) and pyrexia (fever). These signs suggest the possibility of dissemination, and may indicate an immunocompromised patient.

## Diagnosis and Treatment

*An early warning sign should be the nodule which drains but does not respond to antibiotics.* The clinician should take a sample of the exudate for cytology, using a microscope slide smear that is stained for examination by a pathologist. A tissue sample should also be obtained by surgical removal (biopsy) and sent to the pathologist. If these tests are negative, a tissue culture should be taken. Organisms are usually easy to detect in the cat, although this is not so simple with the dog. When dealing with canines, a sample of exudate or tissue should be sent to the Centers for Disease Control in Atlanta, GA, for testing. At CDC, clinicians will run a fluorescent antibody test to identify a case of sporotrichosis when exudate, feces or tissue biopsy and cultures fail to find the organism. As far as treatment is concerned, neither dogs nor cats should receive any drugs which might in any way compromise their immune systems. Nor should glucocorticoids such as prednisone be used.

# Treating Dogs

The infected canine should receive a super-saturated solution of potassium iodide solution (SSKI) at a rate of 40 mg/kg. The animal should then be observed closely for hyper-iodism, which appears as dry and scaly skin, ocular and nasal discharge, vomiting and diarrhea, depression and collapse. When these side-effects occur, the drug must be discontinued and later re-instituted in a more controlled and monitored dose. If necessary, as a result of recurrent adverse reactions to SSKI, there may be some benefit from ketoconazole (Nizoral) and other drugs within this chemical class, according to some investigators. However, this requires taking the medicine with an acid meal (such as tomato juice). The side-effects of ketoconazole use in dogs may include loss of appetite, vomiting, hair loss, and lightening of the haircoat.

# Treating Cats

Even though felines are extremely sensitive to iodine, SSKI therapy should be started at 20 mg/kg, with very careful monitoring for hyper-iodism. Adverse signs include muscle twitching, increased temperature and cardiovascular failure. As in the dog, if complications from SSKI occur, try ketoconazole. This alternative medication also has adverse reactions including liver damage, fever, vomiting, diarrhea and neurological signs.

# Public Health Prognosis

The diagnosis of this disease, particularly in cats, requires the pet owner to make a very difficult decision. Knowing how severely contagious the disease is, the owner should consider euthanasia. That is especially true for people who come in contact with HIV-infected individuals, or those who are taking any sort of immuno-suppressant or chemotherapeutic drugs. For these individuals, there are certainly risks involved in being near a cat with sporotrichosis.

# 7

# ECTOPARASITES

## Scabies

*By Dr. Steven A. Melman, Potomac, Maryland*

Who would ever think that something as small as a mite could cause an itchy skin disease as big as scabies — an ailment that can strike both dogs and their human owners. Scabies, which is more commonly known as "sarcoptic mange," is caused by a mite whose name is longer than the tiny arachnid itself: *Sarcoptes scabieii var. canis*. Whenever veterinarians can't figure out what other parasite (or ectoparasite, as parasites of the flesh are called) could be causing a dog such terrible itchiness, they usually pay close attention to the microscopic mite. In fact, scabies was found to be the seventh most prevalent skin disorder among dogs, according to one survey.

The incidence of scabies can differ from region to region. For example, at my West Coast clinic I see a much higher incidence of sarcoptic mange than at my East Coast site. This observation is supported by colleagues who have witnessed similar regional differences in scabies infections. Aside from seasonal considerations, housing and hygiene also seem to have an effect on the incidence of scabies. The scabies mite lives a full but relatively short life, ranging from only 17 to 21 days. Most of this time is spent on (or in) the skin of the host animal. In fact, a mite without a host is doomed to die within 24 to 36 hours in the average (clean) household. Nevertheless, mites are still pretty picky about what animal they prefer to live on. So it is that the dog-specific mite will likely be found only on the family canine, although in a pinch the mite can take a quick meal from another animal — including a human.

Mites burrow into the skin, where they spend their lives under the top layer of the epidermis (the *stratum corneum*). Problems arise when the host animal experiences a hypersensitivity or allergy to the mite. We know this because:

1) The signs and severity of itching will vary between animals;

2) There is a latent, non-clinical period of up to four weeks before clinical signs appear;

3) Re-exposure to mites causes immediate clinical signs;

4) Itching and nodules can persist despite eradication of mites; and

5) Only a few mites are necessary to cause a reaction.

## Clinical Signs

The cardinal sign of scabies is pruritus (itching). Although there is not an age, breed or sex predisposition, young dogs seem to be more commonly affected — perhaps due to population dynamics, since young dogs socialize more than older ones do. The most common signs of infection are lesions or red bumps on the ear pinnae, extremities and axillae. Many cases progress to generalized scaling, alopecia (hair loss) and crusting with a typical rancid odor.

There is a 10 to 50 percent possibility that other animals in the household may also get hit with the scabies mite, which is why all exposed animals in a household should be treated — regardless of whether or not they have symptoms of scabies. On dogs, the mite seems to take a special liking of certain pressure points such as elbows and hocks. Scabies can become quite serious, progressing to emaciation and eventual death. At the other end of the spectrum are those animals with "scabies incognito." These are animals that are itchy, although they still retain their good coats and show no other clinical signs except that they respond to standard scabies treatment. Lymph nodes are commonly enlarged.

One unusual clinical symptom that is easily demonstrated in the veterinary exam room is a positive "thump" or "pinnal/femoral" reflex. The veterinarian will rub the tip of the patient's ears together so that the skin rubs together. If the patient responds with a thumping reflex of the hindleg, the test is positive. It must be emphasized that this test is merely suggestive, and that many other diseases can cause a positive reaction to the "thump" test! The symptoms of scabies — especially scabies incognito — share a lot in common with other itch-causing ailments such as atopy (inhalant allergy), food allergy, contact allergy, other ectoparasites and skin infections (pyoderma). That puts the heat on the veterinarian to make a careful diagnosis and follow through with appropriate treatment.

## Diagnosis

The best diagnostic test for scabies is a positive skin scraping that will reveal the presence of the mite. Depending upon who is doing the scraping and what sites are selected, the presence of mites is found in only 5 to 20 percent of cases — poor odds by any standards. For this reason, a negative skin scraping is not enough to automatically rule out a diagnosis of scabies. A biopsy is even less likely to turn up signs of mites. Occasionally, fecal flotation will demonstrate mites. At my clinic, the most effective way I diagnose scabies is by beginning treatment, and watching carefully for a positive response. If the patient responds to therapy, then I know that scabies was at least a part of the problem.

## Treatment

All animals that have come into contact with a scabies-infected animal should be treated and kept in isolation until the veterinarian has been able to evaluate the patient's response to the treatment. Ivermectin is the treatment of choice for scabies in dogs other than collies or collie crosses. (For some reason, the drug causes *severe* reactions in collies and their crosses.) Ivermectin, which is administered orally, is preferred to topical therapy for a number of reasons. Pet owners appreciate the fact that it is easy to administer, inexpensive and very effective. Unfortunately, the Food and Drug Administration (FDA) has not approved the use of ivermectin for treatment of scabies in small animals. And while veterinarians still rely on ivermectin for treatment of scabies, it is their responsibility to notify their clients of any risks involved.

Alternative therapy — which *can* be used on collies — includes the use of topical medications such as lime sulfur dips (Lym Dip/DVM), amitraz (Mit-a-ban Upjohn) and phosmet (Paramite/Vet Kem). Unfortunately, dipping is very labor-intense, requiring frequent baths in toxic, bad-smelling chemicals. Often the coat should be clipped to enable the chemical to more effectively reach the affected skin. The clinician should not forget to provide other supportive therapy designed to treat other clinical signs which may be primary or secondary to scabies. Usually this means the simultaneous administration of anti-itch medications. I prefer the use of DermaPet Oatmeal Conditioner, which can be applied to the patient several times daily to relieve itching. Prior to dipping, I prefer the Step 3 treatment method (as described in Chapter 4), which involves the use of a hypo-allergenic shampoo followed by DermaPet Benzoyl Peroxide Plus or Sulfoxydex (DVM) (which also contains sulfur). This will help relieve the itchiness as well as treat and remove the scales and crusts that are often present.

# Flea Control

By Dr. Steven A. Melman, Potomac, Maryland

Sometimes it's hard to keep the Great Outdoors from coming indoors. That's especially true for fleas, which all too often find a way to hop from the comfort of some tall grasses to the luxury of plush carpeting and feathery soft sofa cushions. "Ah, this is the life," you can almost imagine the fleas saying, as they lounge around the house contentedly feeding off whatever warm-blooded restaurant happens by. That's not the way it's supposed to be, but for a lot of pet owners, that's exactly what happens to their homes in the summertime, when the living is easy ... for fleas.

Knowledge is the weapon most lacking in most flea fighters' arsenals. Before attempting to go to war against fleas, the wise pet owner should be aware of the role played by the environment. Of great importance is the temperature and humidity. The optimum comfort zone for fleas is a temperature between 60 to 80 degrees Fahrenheit, and a similar percent humidity. This means that when the temperature and humidity approach these levels, you should have an active, ongoing flea control plan.

## The Life Cycle of Fleas

Female fleas can lay eggs for over a year. Eggs usually are attracted to dark areas, like cracks and crevices indoors or away from light in bushes and high grass. They rarely are seen or recognized in nature. Another stage in the life cycle is called the pupae, in which the immature, non-reproducing flea larva spins a cocoon to protect it from outside elements. The flea egg and pupae are very resistant to standard chemicals normally used in flea control. Only recently have certain Insect Growth Regulators (IGRs) been found effective in killing flea eggs.

It takes four weeks to one year for an egg to develop into an adult breeding flea. The three larval stages and the pupal stage each take as little as one week before a breeding adult emerges. Pyramidal growth occurs and the rate of maturation increases as the environment gets closer to optimum temperature and humidity. The main flea affecting the dog and cat in North America is the cat flea, *Ctenocephalides felis*. Oddly enough, cats usually are asymptomatic carriers, while their canine counterparts often suffer from flea allergy. Because cats are non-allergic to fleas, many authorities refer to the cat as the "Typhoid

Mary" of the flea world.

Fleas can carry a number of diseases, some of which can be contagious and even deadly to man. One of the more benign but aggravating afflictions to which the flea serves as an intermediate host is the dog and cat tapeworm, *Dipylidium caninum*. This tapeworm, which appears as a rice-like segment in the feces, is not believed to be contagious to man (except in one rare reported instance).

## Seek Professional Advice

Generally speaking, you should go to your veterinarian for advice on a difficult infestation. Difficult or recurring cases usually require professional intervention. When one is available, you should seek the assistance of a formally trained dermatology referralist who specializes in problem cases. He or she will guide you in the selection of chemicals and in developing a sound plan. A working knowledge of the flea's life cycle, flea habits and pesticide chemistry are necessary tools in the war against fleas. Your own personality and personal situation (pregnancy, crawling infants, age and personal afflictions) as well as your pet's idiosyncracies will need to be considered in developing an effective flea control plan. The ultimate goal is to select the least toxic and most environmentally sensitive pesticides to safely and effectively deal with your situation.

Remember, an effective flea control program demands a commitment to both product and action. One without the other is not going to do the job, and pet owners should know that. So be sure you not only use the products you buy, but use them *properly*, and aggressively take extra steps to guarantee the house is free of fleas. And always make sure to read the label carefully.

## Chemicals for Indoor and Outdoor Use

Treatment of the house and outdoors demands the use of three different chemical classes: a residual; a quick kill; and an IGR, or insect growth regulator. Use something from each of these different chemical classes simultaneously for best effect. My usual recommendations are:

### Residuals

Any insecticide chosen for outdoor use should be a *residual* chemical, one that is not inactivated easily. One such candidate, for example, is chlorpyrifos (trade name Dursban), a member of the *organophosphate* (OP) chemical class. But remember, Dursban is highly toxic to all vertebrates, including you, your pet and all other friendly animals in the environment, like birds. Cat owners especially should not let their felines near the stuff till it has dried properly. OPs are cholinesterase inhibitors, which is why they were originally developed as nerve gas causing involuntary twitching.

Another class of residual chemicals are the *carbamates*, with the most well-known member being carbaryl. However, carbaryl has been in disfavor with many flea-control experts who claim that fleas have grown resistant to it. Others blame a poor overall flea control plan, and still others say it is a combination of resistance on the part of fleas and poor planning on the part of humans.

### Quick-kills

Botanicals are actually derived from naturally occurring plants, such as chrysanthemums (pyrethins), citrus extracts (d-limonene) and the cube root (rotenone). Pyrethins are the most commonly selected, and they're my recommendation for "on-pet" flea control agents mainly because they can be used daily and are not cholinesterase inhibitors.

However, the same property which makes pyrethins desirable for use on pets indoors—they are quickly inactivated in the environment—poses a major disadvantage when they are used outdoors: they are exquisitely sensitive to sunlight. That's why researchers developed sturdier synthetic botanicals, called *pyrethroids* (such as permethrin). Synthetic botanicals are used both indoors and outdoors, and on pets. Pyrethroids, like their cousins pyrethins, share the quality of decreased toxicity to mammals but also can be residual.

### IGRs

Called "insect growth regulators," these interrupt the maturation process of the baby flea, preventing it from reaching adulthood while not actually killing it. They will soon be licensed for outdoor use. IGRs are generally the least toxic chemical class. Many areas of the United States sprayed an IGR (dimilin) for gypsy moth control. Although dimilin is not yet registered for fleas, it seems to be effective against them. Two other IGRs currently available for "in-home" or "on animal" use are fenoxycarb and methoprene (Precor). Nilar should be available. Methoprene cannot be used outdoors, since it is easily inactivated by sunlight. It is the essential ingredient in a new flea collar which, among other claims, uses the pet as an applicator to its environment. Other IGRs which show much promise will be on the market in the near future.

## Cleaning and Grooming

Careful skin and coat care is fundamental to effective flea control. During flea season, I suggest weekly bathing with a hypoallergenic, moisturizing shampoo like DermaPet Conditioning Shampoo. Hypoallergenic baths should be followed by a pyrethrin dip. A conditioner should be added to the dip to assist in penetration and to keep the coat and skin healthy (See Chapter 4). Take great care to avoid selecting a conditioner/bath oil that contains a synergist (e.g., sesame oil). This might potentiate your dip so that it becomes very deadly to your pet. The conditioner should be used on a daily basis to nourish the coat and skin. If your local pet shop offers grooming services, bring in your dog or cat for bathing, dipping and clipping. A healthy coat and skin is not attractive to fleas.

Pet hair should be clipped somewhat shorter in the flea season to make detection and elimination much easier. That's especially true in regions where ticks and Lyme Disease are a problem. The judicious use of a flea comb on a regular basis will help in identifying an infestation. In fact, if you have brought in your pet for grooming, make sure you use the flea comb on your pet before it leaves the shop, to demonstrate that the groomer has done her job. If you get home and comb your dog again, and discover fleas, you will know that the insects are still in the house, and you can locate the problem.

## Repellents, Sprays and Shampoos

Repellents are a popular — but up until recently, ineffective — group of chemicals. No chemical has been approved by the government as a repellent that is actually effective. Avon Skin-So-Soft has been successfully used as a mosquito and flea repellent for years, on humans. But due to its greasiness and the fact that it is formulated for people, not animals, it is at best unattractive for use on pets. The author designed DermaPet Conditioner as a combination Avon Skin-So-Soft, humectant and emollient for pets. So far, the product has outperformed its expectations.

Pyrethrin sprays can be used safely on a daily basis before the pet goes outside. There are also firms making spray-on hair conditioners that can be used daily to contribute to healthy skin and coat. Some of these products may help to repel fleas.

Although flea and tick collars are the best selling products in the pet industry, they are virtually also the least effective. These products, popular for their convenient usage, are potentially toxic to the pet, its owner and the environment.

Flea shampoo is also vastly overrated, since you must use a quick-killing chemical and leave it on for about 10 minutes. Most shampoos without insecticides will kill fleas in this time. Also, flea shampoos deliver varying concentrations and quantities of pesticide that vary according to the user, the type and quantity of water used, coat thickness, coat length, size of dog and other important variables. Generally speaking, never use a flea shampoo and dip of the same insecticide class.

95

## Other Formulations

There are many formulations to deliver various pesticides to pets. It is outside the scope of this chapter to give justice to all of them. In brief, I do *not* recommend for "on-pet" flea control:

1) the use of systemic pesticides, such as cythioate (Proban), which is a tablet;

2) topically administered fenthion (Pro-Spot);

3) permethrin (Exspot), although I have heard good things about this product for tick control;

4) FBPs (follicle binding polymers) such as Shield, which seem to prolong the breakdown of a non-residual chemical; and

5) microencapsulated products, which decrease the toxicity of residual chemicals. Usually, I prefer frequent use of low-toxicity chemicals over the FBPs and microencapsulated products.

Recent development of "on-animal" growth regulators offers exciting new formulations which I recommend using. Unfortunately, the frequency of use (they have good residual and low toxicity) needed for these mixtures requires the purchase of a second compound for everyday use, unless the user wishes to simply waste the IGR component.

## The Role of Nutrition

I cannot over-emphasize the need for daily brushing and a nutritious diet that will contribute to a healthy coat. If you are not already feeding premium foods to your pet, pick up some sample sizes. Food additives like brewer's yeast, sulfur and garlic have no scientific support for claims as to their effectiveness. In fact, one study showed brewer's yeast and sulfur to be no better than a placebo.

Research done by my daughter in her junior high school prize-winning science project showed that brewer's yeast actually energized live fleas while garlic killed them on contact. Unfortunately, there is no evidence that if ingested, garlic is effective. I am doing research in the field of all-natural flea control, which hopefully will lead to some exciting new and safe products.

Before a pesticide application, turn the house upside down. Clean, mop and vacuum the premises thoroughly. When vacuuming, pay special attention to your pet's favorite areas. Also vacuum under furniture cushions, chairs and beds, and along the walls. Not only does vacuuming suck up renegade fleas and their eggs, larvae and feces. It also picks up dust mites, allergens, and the many other components of house dust.

Some pet owners like to place mothballs in the vacuum cleaner bag. If you do this, throw away the bag *immediately* after the cleaning is done. You should be aware that live fleas can be quite cozy inside the vacuum bag, with all that hair and dust. So be sure the used bag is disposed of in a tightly sealed container. In a severe infestation, you may find steam cleaning of carpets is also necessary. All bed sheets, blankets and comforters—both yours and your pet's—should be laundered, if possible.

Other areas, such as the kitchen, bathroom or enclosed patios, should also be washed with a warm soapy solution. Flea eggs and larvae can live undetected in nooks and cracks until the big day comes and they emerge to feed upon pets and people. A small amount of bleach can be added to hot water as a general disinfectant. Otherwise, you can buy a cleaning agent, or possibly a citrus-based product.

## "Evicting" the Fleas

The house needs to be safely but effectively saturated with a variety of insecticides. The most popular "in-home" anti-flea products today are TRAs (total release aerosols), or "bombs" and "foggers" as they're commonly called. However, if these products are used improperly, they are relatively ineffective in ridding the home of fleas. Bombs do not go through walls or under furniture, and using them may require turning off pilot lights on gas stoves or covering up plastic-based products and houseplants. Don't forget to cover up kitchen utensils.

That's why it is necessary to vacuum and clean first, and remove all sofa or chair cushions and furniture to enable the bomb to function well. This should be followed with a liquid concentrate spray, using chemicals described above, in areas the fogger may not have hit, such as under the furniture.

My recommendations will vary in a home with a pregnant mother and crawling infants. In these situations, you should use a microencapsulated product, in addition to pyrethrins and an IGR. Microencapsulation decreases toxicity, and in many cases prolongs efficacy. Unfortunately, vacuuming may pick up these tiny microcapsules before they attach to fleas. I'll say it again: Anytime you buy a pesticide, *read the label carefully.*

The home should be treated on a monthly basis during the flea season. For regular prevention—and always during an infestation—have a professional exterminator visit the house and talk about what specific tactics can be taken to eliminate flea infestation.

## Treating the Yard

Before wasting time and money spraying your yard with insecticides, you should do a little outdoor cleaning. If the lawn is overgrown, cut it. If dead leaves and other debris are gathering in piles, remove them. A yard free of debris and tall grass is also less likely to be infested with ticks, those carriers of potentially fatal Lyme Disease among other maladies.

You need to "zone off" the yard into two basic areas: the *dead zone* and the *safe zone*.

- **The dead zone**. This is the area of the yard most frequently used. It is here that you need to prevent weeds and high grasses from growing rampant, and prevent excessive moisture such as still water.

- **The safe zone**. Immediately outside the dead zone is the safe zone, where you should maintain the grounds as best as possible.

Both zones need to receive insecticide treatment, as prescribed on the product label. But be warned that a variety of environmental factors can contribute to both the health and hardiness of their residential flea populations, and the effectiveness of the flea-kill products. For example, what if you live on a lake in the South, and your flea-allergic Labrador retriever loves to swim before lazing under the trees or chasing the barn cats around the bushes? You're going to have problems. For those of you whose life is less complicated, there is hope.

Generally, fleas do not love excessive heat or dryness. Nor do they enjoy high altitudes. That means those folks with lakefront homes in temperate climates or humid tropical regions have no choice but to move to the mountains and deserts. Or, they can undertake a vigorous program of flea control. What choice would *you* take? Most likely, you'll be glad to stay put and use outdoor flea-kill remedies. However, unless a product is labeled for use outdoors, it should not be used in the yard.

Consult the daily newspaper, local newscast or The Weather Channel for a long-range weather forecast. If the forecast calls for rain, you shouldn't even think about treating the yard, because rain will simply dilute the chemicals. In cases of infestation, the yard should be treated at two-week intervals three times. Thereafter, maintenance should occur monthly. Small areas may only require a dust product such as diazinon, which is an organophosphate. Homeowners should concentrate their chemical application most heavily in the dead zone, where pets will most likely spend much of their outdoor play time.

In the larger safe zone, owners can use a spray product that requires attachment to a garden hose. But take care to prevent unnecessary dilution with water. That can happen if you remove a finger from the venture orifice, causing dispersal of water.

Some manufacturers of flea-killing yard sprays also claim their products are good for killing ticks, cockroaches, palmetto bugs, ants and sowbugs. Well, why not? And once all the yardwork is done, it's time to pick up the dog at the groomer. But before that, really cautious pet owners may want the extra assurance of knowing their cars are also flea-free. That requires the use of an IGR and a quick-killing pyrethrin. Never use a residual chemical in an automobile. You see, the chemicals can contaminate the ventilation system, and in the enclosed environment of the automobile, the results can be dangerous.

In the end, no program to eliminate fleas will be effective unless it is also comprehensive and takes every possible variable into account. One can never overemphasize the need for proper cleaning, grooming and feeding, as well as regular veterinary checkups. Learn as much as you can about fleas and pesticides. Keep reading articles to find out what is new and try the least toxic methods. Remember that a well-nourished pet with a clean, healthy coat is less likely to develop a serious flea problem.

# Demodex

*By Dr. Linda Medleau, Athens, Georgia*

When mites are around, there are bound to be problems. And in the case of dogs, the trouble starts with large numbers of mites called *Demodex canis*, which are the direct cause of the canine demodicosis skin disease. These tiny arachnids are normal inhabitants on canine skin. Practically all dogs have at least a few, living in the hair follicles and being transmitted to puppies by their mothers. However, the number of mites in the average dog's skin remains relatively low, thanks to the canine immune system. As long as the mites are few in number, no disease is seen. But if the canine immune system is suppressed by some deficiency, stress or disease, the mites may overpopulate their "city on legs" and cause clinical disease.

# Clinical Signs

Demodicosis occurs in two forms: *localized* and *generalized*.

### Localized Demodicosis

Localized demodicosis is the most common form in dogs less than one year old. In this form, the dog develops a few circular or patchy areas of hair loss. Affected skin may be scaly, with either a normal, reddish or grayish color. Lesions are usually seen on the muzzle, around one or both eyes, near the lips, on the head, front legs or trunk. And unless they are also infected, the areas of hair loss are not painful or itchy. While most cases of localized demodicosis resolve themselves within four to eight weeks, some cases progress to the next level.

### Generalized Demodicosis

Generalized demodicosis comes in two varieties, depending on the age of the affected canine: *generalized juvenile-onset demodicosis* and *generalized adult-onset demodicosis*.

Juvenile-onset demodicosis is usually seen in dogs up to one year old. Breeds predisposed to the ailment include the Afghan hound, beagle, Boston terrier, boxer, chihuahua, shar-pei, chow chow, collie, Dalmatian, dachshund, Doberman pinscher, English bulldog, German shepherd, great Dane, old English sheepdog, pointer, pit bull terrier, pug and Staffordshire bull terrier. However, any breed — including mixed breed dogs — can get the disease. Dogs older than one year are more likely to be afflicted with generalized adult-onset demodicosis. Any breed of dog can get it. Because the animals are older, some underlying problem that is affecting the immune system is usually present. This can be a hormonal imbalance (hypothyroidism, hyperadrenocorticism), diabetes mellitus, cancer or treatment with immunosuppressive drugs like steroids. Both forms of generalized demodicosis begin as a localized disease that spreads. Usually there are areas of patchy or diffuse hair loss, and affected skin may also be reddened, grayish, scaly and have bumps or crusts. If the feet are affected, they may be swollen and painful. The dog may be itchy, especially if its skin is also infected. If the skin is badly infected, the dog may have a fever, be depressed and refuse to eat.

# Diagnosis and Treatment

In both localized and generalized demodicosis, the disease is diagnosed by finding demodectic mites in skin scrapings. Because the mites can be hard to find on scrapings taken from the feet, or if the dog's skin is thick, biopsies may be needed to make a diagnosis. If the skin is also infected, swab samples are usually submitted to a diagnostic laboratory in order to identify the invading bacteria.

For *localized demodicosis*, a veterinarian may recommend no treatment at all. That's not so odd, since many cases resolve themselves. Daily applications of benzoyl peroxide shampoos, lotions or creams (2.5 to 3 percent solutions), or benzoyl peroxide gel (five percent) to the lesions will help improve the health of the affected skin. Alternately, a topical product that kills mites can be applied to the lesions once a day. Topicals include rotenone in mineral oil (Canex), benzyl benzoate lotion, and amitraz (Mitaban) — 0.66 ml per 8 oz. water, mixed fresh daily. Localized lesions should be re-checked and re-scraped every two to four weeks. The treatment will continue until the skin scrapes show no mites, and the skin lesions have healed. To help prevent localized demodicosis from advancing into the generalized form, it is important to keep the dog as healthy as possible. This includes making the sure the animal's vaccinations are current, seeing that it is de-wormed, fed a good quality dog food, and kept clear of stressful situations such as kennel boarding or dog shows. Because steroids suppress the immune system, they definitely should not be given to dogs suffering from localized demodicosis, or generalized demodicosis may develop.

For *generalized demodicosis*, treatment can be difficult and expensive. However, the long-term prognosis has improved, and treatment has become less complicated with the advent of amitraz (Mitaban). Even dogs that cannot be completely cured may be kept under control by intermittent treatments continued indefinitely. A hereditary predisposition to juvenile-onset generalized demodicosis is suspected, because certain breeds and lines have an increased tendency to develop the ailment. For this reason, the American Academy of Veterinary Dermatology recommends that any dog developing generalized demodicosis before the age of one be neutered. Estrus or pregnancy may trigger relapses in recovered females, a problem easily avoided with neutering. In dogs with adult-onset demodicosis, the underlying problem should be identified and controlled if possible in order to successfully treat the disease. Steroids should be avoided. Currently, the only treatment for dogs with generalized demodicosis that has won approval from the U.S. Food and Drug Administration is amitraz (Mitaban) at a concentration of 0.025 percent, applied to the body every two weeks. This concentration is prepared by diluting one bottle (10.6 ml) in two gallons of warm water, or one-half bottle (5.3 ml) in one gallon of water immediately before use.

Prior to the first treatment, the haircoat should be clipped with a No. 10 or 15 blade if the dog is medium- or long-haired. Without a clipping, the treatment will not work for these dogs. The animal should be bathed with a shampoo containing benzoyl peroxide to remove scales and crusts and flush out the hair follicles where the mites hide. Then dry the dog with a towel or hair dryer, and apply the freshly prepared Mitaban solution to the animal's body with a sponge until the haircoat and skin are saturated. The entire body, including the face, should be treated. The human bather should wear rubber gloves and protective clothing. The dog should be allowed to air-dry, without getting wet between treatments. Veterinarians will take skin scrapings every two to four weeks in order to monitor the animal's response to the treatments, which should continue for as long as four weeks after the scrapings show no signs of mites. It can take several months for the dog to fully recover, but if the treatments are stopped too early, a relapse will occur.

Concurrent treatment with antibiotics may be necessary if the dog's skin is also infected by a bacteria of some sort. The choice of antibiotic is usually based on culture results. The most common side-effect of the Mitaban treatment is sedation, which is usually mild but may last up to 72 hours. This occurs most often in toy breeds. Some veterinarians have advised using half the recommended concentration for the first two treatments in order to minimize the possible side-effect. Other uncommon side-effects include decreased appetite, excessive drinking and urination, itching, seizures, muscle weakness and, rarely, death.

## Alternative Therapies

Mitaban is much more effective when applied once a week, although it has only been approved for use every two weeks. Consequently, many veterinary dermatologists prefer to treat generalized demodicosis with the approved concentration of 0.025 percent Mitaban, but at weekly intervals. If skin scrapings show increased numbers of mites after four to six treatments, the concentration of Mitaban can be doubled. Demodicosis of the feet is especially difficult to treat, and approved therapy may not be enough. Mitaban can be applied to the feet once or twice during the interval between the whole-body dips. Each treatment should consist of soaking the feet in the Mitaban solution for 10 minutes. These foot soaks have been found most effective when a 0.125 percent concentration (0.63 ml Mitaban per 100 ml water) is used.

An alternative to foot soaks is to apply a solution of 0.5 ml Mitaban in 30 ml of mineral oil to the feet every three days. None of these uses of Mitaban is approved. In some dogs, Mitaban treatment helps relieve or heal the skin lesions, but does not completely eliminate the mites. In these dogs, lesions may be kept in remission by applying Mitaban at two- to eight-week intervals.

What if even weekly treatments with Mitaban fail to resolve the demodicosis? Other treatments for persistent cases of generalized demodicosis in dogs have been described. These treatments are not approved for use in dogs. One such treatment is to use milbemycin (Interceptor), a drug that is only approved for use in dogs as a monthly heartworm and hookworm preventative. For generalized demodicosis, the monthly dosage of Interceptor is doubled and given orally once a day. Treatment is continued two to four weeks after skin scrapings become negative. Side-effects are uncommon, but there have been reports of certain muscle weaknesses that went away once the treatment was stopped. The use of oral ivermectin (0.27 mg/lb/day) also has been effective in many dogs with chronic demodicosis. Treatment is continued until skin scrapings show no mites, plus another two weeks just to be safe. Most dogs recover within two months. However, this unapproved use of ivermectin may result in adverse reactions in dogs (tremors, muscle weakness, dilated pupils, coma and death). Purebred and mixed-bred collies, Shetland sheepdogs, Old English sheepdogs

---

# *Feline Demodicosis*

In cats, demodicosis can be caused by two different *Demodex* mites. It is a rare disease that is often in tandem with an underlying disease such as feline leukemia virus, feline immunodeficiency virus (feline AIDS), or diabete mellitus. Cats can get localized or generalized demodicosis, just like dogs. Localized demodicosis can be seen as patchy areas of hair loss on the eyelids, around the eyes, and on the head or neck. The affected skin may also be reddened, scaly, and crusty. The lesions can be very itchy in some cats, while in others the disease can also cause a waxy ear infection. Generalized demodicosis may involve the head, neck, legs, trunk, flanks, chest and stomach. Usually there is patchy or diffuse hair loss. Affected skin may be reddened, scaly and crusty. Sometimes the skin is also darker in color. The cat may or may not be itchy. The veterinary dermatologist will diagnose the illness by finding mites on skin scrapings or on ear swabs.

### *Treatment*

Although localized demodicosis may spontaneously resolve itself, it can be treated topically with rotenone in mineral oil (Canex) applied to the lesions once a day. In generalized demodicosis, the underlying disease should be identified and treated, if possible. The only approved treatment for generalized demodicosis in cats is a two percent lime sulfur solution, applied topically once a week until skin scrapings are negative. Freshly prepared lime sulfur solution is sponged on the entire body, and the cat is then allowed to air dry. This solution smells terrible (at least until the cat is dry), but it is extremely safe for use on cats and kittens. Other treatments have been employed, but they are not approved for use on felines. These potentially toxic treatments include Mitaban, Paramite and malathion dips.

and Australian shepherds are extremely susceptible to possible adverse reactions from the extra-label use of ivermectin. Signs of side-effects may develop from as early as four to six hours after oral ivermectin's administration, to as long as 10 to 12 hours later. Most dogs will recover within seven to 10 days, but severely depressed and comatose patients may take longer.

Ivermectin is a microfilaricide, so dogs should be evaluated for heartworm disease before it is used. That's because dogs with heartworms may have very severe reactions to ivermectin. Reactions usually occur within one to four hours after administration, and may include vomiting, trembling, breathing difficulties and collapse. Supportive care with intravenous fluids and steroids may be needed if the dog is in shock.

# Cheyletiella or Walking Dandruff

*By Dr. Steven A. Melman, Potomac, Maryland*

Ectoparasites are parasites which live on the skin of animals. The most common ectoparasite is the flea, discussed in a separate article. *Demodex* and *Sarcoptes* are other common ectoparasites, also discussed separately. This article will consider *Cheyletiella*, a common cause of itchy skin disorders. Often called "walking dandruff" because it appears as flakes or scales on the coat of dogs, cats and rabbits, Cheyletiella is caused by the mite *Cheyletiella yasguri* (dogs), *blakeii* (cats) and *parsitovorax* (rabbits) *var. canis*. Before making a diagnosis of any non-seasonal itchy skin disorder and seborrhea, one must rule out *Cheyletiella*. The incidence of this disorder varies from region to region. Because *Cheyletiella* is easily treated by most methods of flea control, it is less prevalent where fleas are a year-round problem. It is more common in *young* animals from animal control facilities, kennels and pet shops, and in breeds that are professionally groomed. Debilitating illnesses, poor hygiene, overcrowding, malnutrition and poor sanitation all predispose animals to infection. It is highly contagious and is zoonotic; that is, it may affect humans. The mites are very large and can be identified easily from skin scrapings. Telltale signs are the hooks on the end of their accessory mouth parts, and legs that end in combs. They live in the stratum corneum (the top layer of skin), although they do not ingest keratin debris but prefer to bite the animal and eat lymph. The mite's life cycle on the host is five to six weeks. The eggs live on hair shafts, where they are not as firmly attached as louse eggs; this is a major difference between lice and *Cheyletiella*. They do not survive well off the host, with survival times similar to scabies (See page 89). As with scabies, itchiness is considered a sign of hypersensitivity or allergy to the mite.

## Clinical Signs

The hallmark of infestation is *scaling* and *pruritus* (itching). Scaling is especially prevalent. One should not conclude that a young cocker spaniel has seborrhea (the breed is predisposed to scaling disorders), before thoroughly checking for *Cheyletiella*. The amount of scaling will vary depending on the color of the coat (white scales are easier to see on a black coat), duration of infestation, overall health, recent bathing and hair length. Should the owner become affected, it is important to note that the mites can live on humans. The characteristic lesion in humans is an erythematous papule (red inflamed bump). It is also important to note that some animals may be asymptomatic carriers; that is, they do not get itchy. In such cases, the animal may live with a symptomatic pet or be owned by someone who has been referred to a dermatologist. This demonstrates the need to treat all contact animals.

## Diagnosis and Treatment

The best diagnostic method is direct visual examination of mites. They can be seen with a magnifying glass, obtained by skin scrape, acetate tape smears and flea comb preparations. Another method is treating a suspected carrier and having the clinical signs disappear.

Eliminating *Cheyletiella* is harder than was once believed. Although more prevalent in non-seasonal flea areas where they are controlled by flea control products, they cannot be eliminated using only flea shampoos, sprays or powders. Successful therapy usually involves a six- to eight-week organized plan of deliberate action, including the following. Again, **all contact animals must be treated**.

1. All long- and medium-haired dogs and cats should have their coats clipped. This mechanically removes mites and eggs which might otherwise be difficult to remove or eliminate with treatment.

2. All dogs and cats should be bathed in a hypo-allergic conditioning shampoo to remove scales. DermaPet Low Antigen Conditioning Shampoo, Hypo-Allergenic Conditioning Shampoo and Mycodex HA Shampoo are my favorite products for this job.

3. As with scabies, ivermectin is my treatment of choice for *Cheyletiella* in

cats, rabbits and dogs other than collies or collie crosses. For some reason, *ivermectin causes severe reactions in collies and their crosses, and should never be given to them.* All contact animals should be treated or isolated until treatment response has been evaluated. Ivermectin is preferred to topical therapy for various reasons. It is easy to administer, inexpensive and very effective. Unfortunately, it has not been approved by the FDA for treating scabies or cheyletiellosis in small animals.

4. Topical therapy can be used at least for the first two treatments (one week). Often puppies are being treated, so different strategies must accommodate different scenarios. Generally, lime sulfur and pyrethrins are the most benign and acceptable agents for treating puppies, lactating or pregnant females, adults and other chemically sensitive animals.

5. Environmental treatment should be instituted. Wash all bedding, including the owner's. Keep the animal out of the bedroom for at least two weeks after beginning therapy. Vacuum and clean. Use a method of household flea control with insecticidal agents other than insect growth regulators as described in the Flea Control article (See page 92). Discard all brushes and combs used on the pet.

# 8

# IMMUNOLOGIC DISEASES

## Overview

*by Dr. Bruce L. Hansen, Springfield, Virginia*
*and Dr. Robert M. Schwartzman, Philadelphia, Pennsylvania*

I n all animals, the immune system's function is to protect the body from disease. The healthy immune system largely accomplishes this through the workings of two internal components — the *humoral system* and the *cell mediated immune system* — which work together to eliminate bacteria, viruses, parasites and even cancerous cells. Some knowledge of how the immune system does this with such amazing efficiency and effectiveness is primary to understanding the various immune-related problems that can arise and leave our pets feeling completely miserable and sick.

### The Humoral System

The Humoral System is mainly made up of white blood cells, called B lymphocytes, which produce *antibodies*. Antibodies (immunoglobulin) are proteins that can bind and remove *antigens* (foreign proteins) such as bacteria, viruses, parasites or fungi. There are several classes (based on size and shape) of antibodies, with each having a specific function. In dogs and cats, the primary antibody or immunoglobulin classes are *immunoglobulin class G* (abbreviated as *IgG*), *immunoglobulin class M* (or *IgM*), *immunoglobulin class A* (or *IgA*), and *immunoglobulin class E* (or *IgE*). Each antibody is very specific, formed to attack and bind only to a specific antigen. For example, an antibody to the deadly parvovirus will bind only to the parvovirus, and not to other bacteria or viruses.

•*IgG/IgM*. The major biological function of the class G immunoglobulins (IgG) is to help remove bacteria, viruses and fungi. Antibodies of the class M (IgM) also have the primary biological function of binding to and removing bacteria, viruses and fungi. However, IgM is the *first* class of antibody formed in an immune response, and therefore it takes up the frontline defense until the more precise and effective IgG type antibody can be produced by the body.

•*IgA*. The main job of IgA antibodies is to inactivate bacteria, viruses and toxins in special areas of the body such as the gastrointestinal tract and mucosal surfaces (for example, the nose, mouth, urinary tract) before these potentially harmful agents can invade the body.

•*IgE*. One of the functions of the IgE antibody is to attack parasites, such as roundworms. However, it is mainly known as the "allergy antibody" for its supposed role in allergic reactions (which will be explained in more detail later on).

### The Cell Mediated Immune System

The Cell Mediated Immune System relies principally upon a type of white blood cell called the *T lymphocyte*. When it encounters antigens, the T lymphocyte produces and secretes large amounts of a protein which regulates inflammation. The inflammation serves to "signal the cavalry," attracting various types of white blood cells that maim, engulf, destroy and eliminate the unwanted foreign protein.

In addition, the T lymphocyte aids the work of another white blood cell, the *B lymphocyte*. If either of these two types of lymphocyte cells are unable to jointly and effectively eliminate antigens, it results in what is known as an *immunodeficiency*. In the human body, a deficiency of a subtype of this cell (T-4 Helper) is found in human AIDS virus. This is an example of an immunodeficiency.

# The Problems that Plague Our Pets

Before diving into a description of the immune-related problems that can affect pets, it is necessary to begin with a few basic definitions:

### Immunologic Diseases

When veterinarians and medical practitioners speak about *immunologic diseases*, they are referring to an entire assortment of diseases caused by hypersensitivity and autoimmunity.

### Hypersensitivity

A healthy immune system is designed to quickly encounter and eliminate any invading foreign proteins, such as bacteria. However, in some cases the immune system will overreact in responding to the antigen. Instead of simply "cleansing" the body of antigens, the immune system will go well beyond what was necessary and actually cause damage to the animal body it was protecting. This condition is called *hypersensitivity*.

### The Allergic Diseases

In veterinary medicine, the hypersensitivity conditions we encounter are known as *the allergic diseases*. This category of problems includes allergic inhalant dermatitis (atopy), food allergy, flea allergy (See Chapter 7), and contact allergy.

### Autoimmunity

On rare occasions, the immune system doesn't attack foreign proteins, but mistakenly *attacks its own body*! This is termed *autoimmunity*.

### The Autoimmune Diseases

In veterinary medicine, a group of autoimmune diseases we occasionally encounter are categorized as *the pemphigus diseases*, (pemphigus foliaceus, pemphigus vulgaris, pemphigus erythematosus, and pemphigus vegetans). Other autoimmune diseases are *bullous pemphigoid*, and *systemic* and *discoid lupus erythematosus*.

## The Allergic Diseases

### Atopy

In allergic inhalant dermatitis, it is believed that antibodies (generally of the IgE class) attach to a skin cell called the *mast cell*. Connected together, these antibodies (and their attached mast cells) encounter the specific foreign protein they are designed to target (such as ragweed pollen), bind to it and cause the mast cell to break apart. The dying mast cell releases tremendous amounts of chemicals, including histamines, proteins and enzymes which then cause the inflammation that starts the allergic reaction. Veterinarians have at their disposal two tests that can help determine whether the skin disease making the patient so uncomfortable is caused by allergic inhalant dermatitis (or what is also called a *hypersensitivity* to inhalant allergens):

• The first possible procedure is to run **blood tests** (*in-vitro testing*) such as the ELISA and the RAST tests. Both the ELISA (enzyme-linked immunosorbent assay) and the RAST (radioallergosorbent test) tests measure the specific levels of IgE to the various suspected offending allergens. If, for example, an animal is allergic to ragweed, you can expect to find very high levels of the ragweed-specific IgE in the body. It would be these high levels of IgE that lead to the allergic reactions.

• The gold standard for identifying inhalant allergies is the **intradermal skin test** (*in-vivo testing*). This involves injecting small amounts of potential allergens into the skin, and watching for a definite reaction. If an animal is allergic to a specific allergen, it will cause the breakup of numerous mast cells. Because the allergen is trapped within the skin with nowhere to "spread out," the subsequent "allergic reaction" remains localized and is manifested by a red welt. The angry red welt usually indicates that the animal has a hypersensitivity to whatever allergen was injected.

There are advantages and disadvantages of both testing methods:

• Blood tests are easy to perform, requiring a quick draw of blood and an overnight shipment to a laboratory. Better yet, the blood test results are unaffected by the presence of a severe skin disease. However, dogs that have been exposed to numerous parasites (remember that one of IgE's main functions is to fight parasites) such as fleas or worms, have developed high levels of all types of IgE — this may in some cases interfere with the test. Fortunately, with proper interpretation by experts at the laboratory, the test can give good results.

• Skin testing can be influenced by many medications the animal is receiving, or by severe skin disease. It also requires that the veterinarian keep a stock of expensive antigens on hand. Finally, the skin test is technically a much more difficult test for the veterinarian to interpret. However, when properly used the intradermal skin test gives very accurate results.

• Positive results of both skin testing and blood testing serve only to alert the veterinarian to the fact that the animal has a hypersensitivity to that specific allergen. The tests do not indicate whether or not the hypersensitivity is actually causing any of the allergic symptoms in the pet. For example, you may be living in Great Britain when you get your dog allergy tested and discover that the animal is allergic to ragweed.

But since there is no ragweed in Great Britain, your dog's allergic symptoms must be caused by something other than ragweed.

Therefore, it is of utmost importance that great care and meticulous attention be directed first at ruling out all other possible causes of itchy skin disease (such as food allergy, flea allergy or infections). In many cases, referral to a veterinary dermatologist may be in the best interest for you and your pet.

### Food Allergies

The exact mechanism behind what causes food-allergic symptoms is still poorly understood. Furthermore, there are no accurate definitive tests for documenting food allergy except for feeding a *hypoallergenic diet trial* for a period of 21 days or longer. A hypoallergenic diet demands feeding the animal a protein source which it does not normally eat (such as lamb, venison or horse meat) along with a starch or carbohydrate that is not normally consumed (such as rice or potatoes) — with no treats or table scraps at all!

Intradermal skin tests and blood tests (ELISA and RAST) are extremely unreliable as far as food allergies are concerned. If the dog's itching and skin disease disappear while the pet is being fed the hypoallergenic diet, the animal is then returned to its old diet. If the itch quickly returns with the old diet, a diagnosis of a probable food allergy is made.

### Allergic Contact Dermatitis

Hair usually serves as a wonderful protective armor against the skin's prolonged contact with a potential allergen, such as poison ivy. However, allergic contact dermatitis can occur on the sparsely haired areas of the belly and in between the pads of the feet. Allergic contact dermatitis can be identified by *provocative exposure* (exposing the animal to the suspected contact allergen and waiting for the skin rash to appear). Another method is *patch testing*, in which a suspected allergen is minced and mixed with petrolatum or petroleum jelly before being taped to a clipped area on the pet. The "patch" is left undisturbed on the animal for 48 hours. The bandage is then removed and the skin examined for the presence of a positive-reaction welt.

# The Autoimmune Diseases

Diseases caused by the body's own immune system attacking itself (autoimmunity) can be very severe and even life-threatening. Diagnosing these diseases is very difficult. Quite often a diagnosis is made based upon the characteristic appearance of lesions, and by microscopic examination of skin tissue obtained through a skin biopsy. Various skin ailments — including autoimmune skin diseases — can be identified through a biopsy because they cause specific microscopic patterns of inflammation. However, only certain areas of the skin disease will show this "diagnostic" pattern of inflammation. Therefore, extreme care should be taken by the veterinarian in selection of proper biopsy sites. In many cases, this step may need to be performed by a veterinary dermatologist with the biopsy slide read by a veterinary dermatopathologist.

Other laboratory tests that can be used in the diagnosis of autoimmune skin disorders include direct immunofluorescence and the use of special stains (immunoperoxidase). In these tests, skin biopsies are treated with fluorescein, or special peroxidase stains, that attach to the antibodies in the skin that are causing the autoimmune disease. If the biopsy slide glows with fluorescence, or is stained with peroxidase stains, an autoimmune skin disease is suspected, with the location of the fluorescence or peroxidase stain within the skin serving as a clue to identifying the particular autoimmune disease. However, severely inflamed skin from a variety of skin diseases can give "false positive" readings suggestive of autoimmune disease. Therefore, these tests should be interpreted in conjunction with the skin biopsy and chemical history.

The *antinuclear antibody test* is a blood test used to diagnose suspected cases of systematic lupus erythematosus (SLE). This very disease destroys large numbers of cells, releasing heavy amounts of proteins from normally well-protected cell nuclei. As more and more of these proteins come in contact with the immune system, the body begins to create antibodies designed to destroy the nuclear proteins. If the antinuclear antibody test turns up a large amount of these anti-nuclear antibodies, in conjunction with clinical signs such as skin and kidney disease or arthritis, a diagnosis of systemic lupus erythematosus can be made.

## No Easy Solutions

Because of the complexity of the immune system and our relative ignorance of this function, immunologic diseases can be difficult to diagnose and even more difficult to control. Continuing research will help us uncover and understand the exact causes of immunologic diseases, and hopefully give us more information in order to diagnose, treat, cure and prevent all those problems that are giving our companion animals so much misery.

# Inhalant Allergy (Atopy)

*A version of the following article appeared in Groom and Board (August 1992)*

*By Dr. Steven A. Melman, Potomac, Maryland*

Laymen call them *allergies*. Scientists refer to them as *Type I hypersensitivities*. Whichever term is used, they are the most common cause of skin diseases in small animals, and arguably the most common cause for concern among pet-care professionals' clients. The most common causes of allergies are fleas, pollen, environmental substances, other animals, and foods. Each type of allergy is associated with numerous symptoms and secondary problems, but the allergic reaction usually causes the animal to scratch, rub, lick, chew or bite at its skin. Common complications include hot spots, skin infections, hair loss and ear infections. Unlike humans, animals rarely cough, sneeze or suffer asthma due to allergies.

Although allergies cannot be cured, they often can be controlled. One fundamental step in controlling any allergy is to identify the cause of the allergic reaction—and then avoid it. However, it may not be easy to avoid the allergen when the substance is in the air we breathe. Therefore, frequent bathing to remove that substance is the next best option. DermaPet Conditioning Shampoo, Mycodex HA (SmithKline Beecham and Norden) and Allergroom (Virbac) are three examples of hypo-allergenic shampoos currently on the market.

Once the allergic reaction has begun, most experts agree that short-acting cortisone-type drugs usually are the most effective non-specific, anti-inflammatory, anti-itch medications. However, cortisone has many side-effects, including an increase in thirst, urination and appetite as well as a decrease in immune response. Antihistamines have been ineffective as treatments for canine allergies, with less than a 30 percent response rate with clemastine (Tavist) and even less with other types. Omega 3 and omega 6 fatty acid supplements have been effective at reducing itching in about 10 percent of cases. Most of the subjects described briefly in this section are extensively covered elsewhere in this book.

## Atopy

Sometimes referred to as allergic inhalant dermatitis or hay fever, atopy occurs in dogs and cats that are hereditarily predisposed to developing antibodies (immunoglobulin E or IgE) to normal environmental proteins. Under normal circumstances, antibodies are protective. However, in the case of atopy, the antibodies have a detrimental effect when a hypersensitivity forms. In the allergic patient, IgE antibodies interact with normal environmental proteins, called "antigens." These include the pollen from plants, trees, grass and weeds as well as house dust, animal dander and molds. This interaction leads to the allergic reaction. In dogs and cats, for example, the allergic reaction typically consists of inflammation and itching.

In humans, the inhalation of an antigen (pollen) triggers the allergic reaction. Signs in the upper respiratory tract include sneezing, coughing and asthma. Dogs and cats also may inhale antigens, but academics argue that antigens on their skin and coat may actually be the most important cause of allergic reactions. Many logical facts support this theory:

---

## *Treating "Hot Spots"*

"Hot spots" are localized areas of self-induced trauma that have become secondarily infected. They usually are moist due to licking and/or weeping (exudation), and hot due to inflammation, itching, irritation and infection. A certain amount of obsessive-compulsiveness overtakes the dog, as if it were trying to put out a fire at that site. Although no one knows for sure, hot spots definitely occur most often in atopic animals and/or as a result of an insect (usually a flea) bite. Here is the treatment I recommend for "uncomplicated" hot spots:

● Use a No. 40 blade to remove all hair around the infected lesion. Be sure to clip down to the skin.

● Bathe the entire animal with a hypoallergenic shampoo to remove all possible antigens.

● Apply a benzoyl peroxide shampoo [*DermaPet Benzoyl Peroxide, Mycodex BP (SmithKline Beecham and Norden), Pyoben (Virbac) and Oxidex (DVM)*] to the affected area, and let the suds sit for a minimum of 5 to 10 minutes. Benzoyl peroxide will reduce the itching sensation, flush out the hair follicles, kill the *staphylococcus* bacteria and dry the lesion. As with all pet dermatological formulations, you should use only benzoyl peroxide preparations designed for dogs. Human products are much stronger and often cause bad reactions. See Chapter 4 (*Shampoo Therapy*) for more information.

● If fleas are present, administer a pyrethrin flea dip and practice environmental flea control methods.

In some cases, the treatments described above fail to yield the expected, relatively quick results. The judicious use of short-acting systemic (oral and/or injectable) corticosteroids, such as prednisone, may be necessary to speed recovery.

"Complicated" hot spots may require further treatment, or a veterinary workup to determine the exact cause of the problem. Certain dog breeds, especially golden retrievers, tend to develop deeply infected hot spots that may require an additional three-week antibiotic treatment.

---

• Dogs and cats respond to pollen allergies with skin diseases.

• Dogs and cats do not wear protective clothing and have not practiced frequent bathing, so they literally wear normal environmental proteins/pollen on their bodies. This can be the source of antigens for the animals themselves or for others who may be allergic to these substances.

• Because skin is the target of the allergic reaction in dogs and cats, and because they wear antigens on their coats, it is only logical to assume that animals absorb antigens through the skin.

• Most veterinary dermatologists recommend that atopic dogs be bathed frequently to remove these antigens. In fact, most human allergists recommend the same for their patients because a pet often serves as a reservoir for antigens.

## Clinical Signs

• The clinical signs of atopy usually appear in pets when they are between one and three years old. Somewhere between 10 and 30 percent of a clinical population will have atopy.

• It is well-known that certain breeds of dogs are predisposed to atopy. While other breeds seem less likely to have this condition, promiscuous breeding seems to have allowed some breeds to catch up. Breeds with an increased incidence of atopy (in the approximate order of relative risk) include: boxers, golden retrievers, West Highland white terriers, Dalmatians, shar-peis, cairn terriers, Scottish terriers, Lhasa apsos, Boston terriers, Sealyham terriers and wire-haired fox terriers. Cocker spaniels and German shepherd dogs are newly recognized as having an increased incidence of atopy. Doberman pinschers, German short-haired pointers and poodles have a decreased incidence of atopy. Poodles, cocker spaniels and German shepherds may appear on either list, depending on where the study is done; this is due to regional variations in breeding. Boxers and German shepherds appear to have an increased incidence of food allergies.

• Dogs with atopy as a result of *pollen* may itch all over, but the itching usually is localized in certain areas. Most often, the face, feet, front legs, ears and armpits are affected.

•The typical *flea-bite hypersensitivity* does not affect the face or front of the animal's body. Lesions caused by fleas most commonly are located above the tail, progressing down the back of the legs and toward the head like a three-dimensional arrow. About half of dogs with atopy also are allergic to fleas.

•Dogs with *food hypersensitivity* do not have lesions in any one typical location. However, cats with food allergies typically have lesions distributed around the head.

## Ear Problems

*Otitis externa*, defined as inflammation of the external ear, can occur in one ear or both as a result of allergies. Approximately 50 percent of atopic dogs have external ear infections; in about five percent, ear problems may be the only sign present. In such cases, ears often are red, waxy, itchy and/or swollen. Occasionally, they ooze as a result of a secondary infection. Treatment always involves controlling the underlying allergy and cleansing the area. Often, a prescription containing a mild corticosteroid preparation is necessary to "douse the fire."

There are many *otic cleansers* on the market. The basic principle is to acidify the ear canal, thus making it undesirable for the growth of yeast or bacteria; and to dry it, thus eliminating any material and moisture that may be present. Otic products containing chlorhexidine (Nolvasan) recently were recalled by the Food and Drug Administration because they cause ear damage in animals that do not have an intact ear (tympanic) membrane — a common complication with ear problems. Another common component of ear cleansing solutions, salicylic acid, has been implicated as an *ototoxicant.* Look for a product that contains acetic acid, boric acid and no alcohol, such as DermaPet Ear/Skin Cleanser.

## Lick Granulomas

Also known as *acral lick dermatitis*, lick granulomas are localized areas of thickened, irritated, inflamed and often ulcerated skin. They usually occur as a result of an obsessive-compulsive disorder, and are most commonly found on the dorsum of the feet, usually the carpus or tarsus. Golden retrievers and Labrador retrievers seem to be predisposed breeds. Allergies seem to be a predisposing factor. Most commonly, these lesions are infected and require long-term treatment with antibiotics. Topical therapy with benzoyl peroxide shampoos is helpful at reducing both the infection and irritation. The underlying cause must be diagnosed and treated.

Often, standard therapy is ineffective, and this leads some investigators to use anti-depressants such as Prozac and Elevil. This therapy is based on work by Judith Rappaport at the National Institutes of Health. She pioneered the use of these drugs in the treatment of obsessive-compulsive disorders (OCDs) such as trichotillomania (a hair pulling OCD) and successfully worked on a group of dogs with lick granulomas. I have had success at the Animal Dermatology Clinics in using these drugs to treat lick granulomas, other OCDs including tail chasing disorders and non-specific pruritic disorders.

## Skin Infections

Also called *pyodermas*, skin infections are not uncommon complications associated with allergy-related skin diseases. They usually are caused by *Staphylococcus* bacteria, which invade the hair follicle. Topical benzoyl peroxide shampoo preparations, as described in the section on hot spots, should be used. In addition, antibiotics should be prescribed for at least three weeks, or seven to 10 days after all signs of infection are gone.

## Food Allergies

Food allergies are among the most overdiagnosed and overtreated conditions in veterinary medicine. Briefly, the best way to diagnose a food allergy is to feed the pet an exclusive diet, such as cooked lamb and long-cooked rice, for three weeks. All treats, supplements or chewable medications must be avoided during this period. If the signs disappear during this period but return soon after the pet resumes its former diet, then the diagnosis of primary food allergy can be made.

In the phenomenon known as *priming*, one antigenic substance combines with another to initiate the allergic reaction. For example, I know a person who had no allergic reaction to sleeping on a feather pillow, living with his cat or eating beef during January — when there was no pollen in the air. In August, when ragweed pollen was present, he reached his allergic threshold and had an allergic reaction to the pillow, cat and beef. He was primed by the ragweed. Food allergy can be either primary or secondary.

I recommend feeding non-specific hypoallergenic diets to animals with food-related allergies.

## Diagnosis

Identifying the specific antigen that triggers the allergic reaction requires careful and somewhat expensive testing, preferably by a veterinarian who has received some postdoctoral training regarding allergies. *Intradermal skin testing* remains the gold standard among such tests. Because it requires a great degree of skill and training, it usually is offered by an individual who operates a referral dermatology practice. Alternative blood tests, such as ELISA or RAST tests, are widely available to all veterinarians and often are selected for convenience or other reasons. These tests are less reliable than intradermal skin testing for many reasons, including the fact that they batch antigens rather than test them individually. Also, there are many more false positive results from blood tests. Blood tests to diagnose food allergies are especially unreliable. At my practices, we use 54 specific antigens selected for their geographic uniqueness in our intradermal skin test kit.

## Other Treatments

Another treatment is *hyposensitization*, the administration of a series of injections containing antigens as determined by skin tests. Although this is the best method to control atopy, it is only 60 to 85 percent successful, depending on your criteria for success. These injections must be given throughout the lifetime of the pet. Unlike humans' allergies, pets' allergies seem to worsen over time. Another alternative is shampoo therapy using hypoallergenic products designed for pets such as DermaPet Conditioning Shampoo. Although many all-natural pet shampoos — with ingredients such as oatmeal, aloe vera, melaleuca, pennyroyal oil or eucalyptus oil — help reduce itching, they are not hypoallergenic and should not be used frequently. Human shampoos should be avoided because they have a bad effect on pets' skin. They often cause flaking, or burn the epidermis.

It is important to remember that pets' skin is very different from humans' skin. Pets have compound follicles, with multiple hairs coming out of each pore, whereas humans have simple follicles, with a single hair per pore. In addition, pets' skin is much thinner (perhaps because it is protected by hair) and has a higher pH (6.6 on average for dogs vs. 5.6 for humans). Pets have sweat glands only in the pads of their feet and on the bridge of their noses. Pets have sebaceous glands all over their bodies, while humans have them primarily on their faces.

In conclusion, it is important to realize that pets are unique, different from humans in many ways. Although they are susceptible to similar diseases, they suffer different symptoms. Because pets are fundamentally different, they require many medications and shampoos designed specifically for them.

# Occurrence of Food Allergy in Dogs And Cats

*By Dr. Kevin P. Byrne, Urbana, Illinois*

Nobody really knows how common food allergies are in dogs and cats. Some veterinary dermatologists speculate that only one percent of the total dog and cat populations suffer from food allergies, while others say that food allergies are the second most common allergy afflicting pets. The real problem is that there is no agreement on when pets should undergo a "hypoallergenic diet trial," a technique commonly used to root out the allergy-causing ingredient in the diet. To further complicate things, it is common for an allergy sufferer to be plagued by more than one offending substance. So if a skin test for inhalant allergies (atopy) shows significant results, a diet trial may never be done — even though the pet may also have food allergy.

Yet another complicating factor is that there are no symptoms which point exclusively to a food allergy. For example, a pet's itchiness (pruritus) can be either a food allergy or a hypersensitivity to flea and mite bites. If you get rid of the fleas, you may lower the animal's "pruritic threshold" to the point that they are not itching anymore, and so they appear to be "cured." But the food allergy is still there, although its signs may be obscure. Food allergy may also manifest itself as a gastrointestinal upset, such as diarrhea or vomiting. Fortunately, this symptom is more common in people than in dogs and cats.

A common misconception is to lump all abnormalities associated with food under the heading of "food allergy." Diarrhea, pruritus, or other signs related to food may not have a true allergic origin, but may instead be caused by other types of food sensitivity. Here are a few terms that can help you understand some of the possible causes for "after-dinner" problems:

• **Food allergy** or **food hypersensitivity** is described as an immunologic reaction (involving the immune system) resulting from a food or food additive (discussed below).

• An **Anaphylactoid reaction** to food is "anaphylaxis-like," meaning that it involves the immune system, *but does not involve the production of allergic* *antibodies by the patient.* Nevertheless, the body releases other irritating substances that can cause the same symptoms of an allergy. For example, the chemical makeup of certain foods can generate adverse anaphylactoid reactions by causing the body to release histamine. When tissues are exposed to histamine, they become inflamed — leading to pain, pruritus, or gastrointestinal upset. There is also a wide array of foods which actually contain high levels of histamine, such as fermented cheeses, sausage, pig liver, spinach, canned tuna and mackerel. Some foods that don't contain histamine can nevertheless cause the body to release histamine. Examples of these include egg whites, shellfish, strawberries, chocolate, fish, alcohol, and tomatoes.

Certain food additives have been known to cause anaphylactoid reactions in humans, and these same substances are also used in certain pet foods. This list includes azo dyes, sodium bisulfite, BHA/BHT, spices, sodium alginate, guar gum, and propylene glycol. Anaphylactoid reactions to food additives are uncommon, and so you need not worry that your pet will automatically have problems just because you see these ingredients on the pet-food label. However, if your pet is having a persistent problem that seemingly can't be solved, you may try to look at these food additives.

• **Food intolerance** is an abnormal response to food that does not involve the immune system. A common example of food intolerance in humans is the diarrhea and intestinal discomfort caused by the inability to digest lactose (milk sugar). A similar condition can occur in adult dogs and cats that drink milk. Digestive disorders may serve to hide a food allergy, because most veterinarians would first consider other causes of stomach upset (such as parasitism, infectious diseases or poisoning) long before they would turn their suspicions on a food allergy as the true culprit.

## How Food Allergy Develops

It was once believed that the digestive tract was a barrier to substances large enough to cause allergy. Only digestion products such as simple sugars, amino acids, fatty acids, vitamins and minerals were believed able to cross this barrier. The only exception to the rule was the "leaky" digestive tract of the newborn child, which allowed the absorption of colostrum from "mother's milk." This colostrum provided antibodies to protect the child. Our views on the permeability of the intestinal tract have changed dramatically. We now know that the intestinal tract is not as impermeable as was once believed. We've discovered that the intestinal tract of both newborns and adults allows the passage of large food molecules (called "macromolecules") that are sizable enough to be allergenic.

There are several ways that food macromolecules can invade the body. One is by slipping through the spaces between the cells that line the intestine (the intestinal epithelial cells). Another way is by the processes of pinocytosis ("cell-drinking") or phagocytosis ("cell-eating") by the intestinal epithelial cells themselves. In other words, potential allergens can get into the body either by leaking between cells or by actually being ingested by the cells. Yet another way for the food macromolecules to get into the body is through the work of special types of tissues called lymphoid tissues, which are located in areas of the body (such as the intestinal tract) that are exposed to the outside environment. (As unusual as it may sound, the insides of the stomach and intestines are considered to be exterior to the bloodstream and other internal organs, though it is a long way from the mouth.)

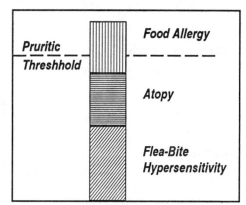

These tissues contain cells called lymphocytes that are responsible for determining whether or not molecules are foreign to the body. One specific type of lymphoid tissue found in the intestinal tract is the "Peyer's-patch," which samples substances inside the intestinal tract. To do this it actually has to carry macromolecules from "outside" the body into the bloodstream. If the

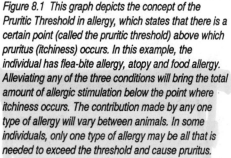

Figure 8.1 *This graph depicts the concept of the Pruritic Threshold in allergy, which states that there is a certain point (called the pruritic threshold) above which pruritus (itchiness) occurs. In this example, the individual has flea-bite allergy, atopy and food allergy. Alleviating any of the three conditions will bring the total amount of allergic stimulation below the point where itchiness occurs. The contribution made by any one type of allergy will vary between animals. In some individuals, only one type of allergy may be all that is needed to exceed the threshold and cause pruritus.*

macromolecules are from a substance that is foreign to the body, such as food, the lymphocytes will produce antibodies against the food macromolecules. And finally, food macromolecules can escape into the body if an individual has a disease that damages the intestinal tract and causes it to "leak." So you see, there are a number of ways the food allergens can gain entry to the body.

Now that we know that allergens can get into the body easily, we have to wonder why every dog or cat doesn't have food allergy. Well, if the ability of potential allergens to cross the intestinal tract was all that's needed to produce food allergy, then every dog, cat and human would probably fall prey to food allergies. Perhaps fortunately, the production of an allergic state ("hypersensitivity") requires that the individual produce an immune reaction that is *excessive* to the allergen. It is this excessive reaction that causes disease.

In food allergy there are several types of hypersensitivity which can occur: Type I, Type III, and Type IV.

## Type I Hypersensitivity

When food molecules (called allergens) gain entry to the body, they are exposed to the lymphoid tissues. Cells in these tissues will produce antibodies called IgE antibodies. These antibodies will attach themselves to two types of cells — called mast cells and basophils. The next time the dog or cat eats that specific food, the allergens are absorbed as before, but now the allergens bind to the IgE antibodies attached to cells. When this occurs, the mast cells and basophils are "turned-on" and release histamine and other substances (mediators). It is this release of histamine and other mediators that causes the clinical signs of itching and redness. This is the most common type of hypersensitivity seen with food allergy and can occur immediately, or take as long as 12 to 24 hours following ingestion of the food.

| Foods Rich In Histamine |
| --- |
| Fermented cheeses |
| Dry pork and beef sausage |
| Pig's liver |
| Canned tuna |
| Meats |
| Spinach |

Table 8.1

## Type III Hypersensitivity

In this type of hypersensitivity, the food allergens bind to antibodies of the IgG type which are in the blood. When allergen binds to these antibodies they can form clusters of allergen-antibody. These clusters have the ability to cause inflammation when they become trapped in small blood vessels and capillaries. This type of hypersensitivity is a rare cause of food allergy.

| Common Histamine-Releasing Foods |
| --- |
| Egg whites |
| Shellfish |
| Chocolate |
| Fish |
| Alcohol |
| Strawberries |
| Tomatoes |

Table 8.2

## Type IV Hypersensitivity

In this type of hypersensitivity, food allergens bind not to a type of antibody, but to a particular type of lymphocyte called the "$T_{dh}$ cell." When binding occurs, this lymphocyte releases substances called lymphokines that induce inflammation in the tissue where the binding occurs. This type of hypersensitivity takes longer to take place, up to 72 hours following ingestion of the food, and so has been called "delayed-type hypersensitivity." In normal individuals

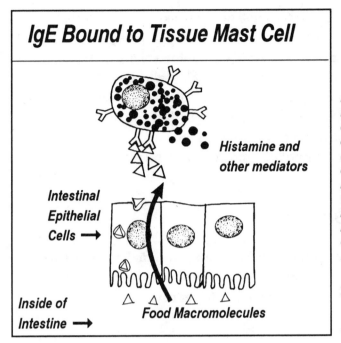

## IgE Bound to Tissue Mast Cell

**Histamine and other mediators**

**Intestinal Epithelial Cells** ➞

**Inside of Intestine** ➞

**Food Macromolecules**

*Figure 8.2 This drawing depicts how food macromolecules are able to enter the body from the intestinal tract due to the process of phagocytosis (cell-eating) by the intestinal epithelial cell. Once inside the body, the macromolecules bind to specific IgE, which are bound to mast cells (or basophils). Binding "turns on" the mast cell to release histamine and other mediators of inflammation. Redness and itchiness of the skin, or "GI" problems, result. (Figure adapted from Tizard, Ian. Veterinary Immunology, an Introduction, 4th Ed., 1992, W.B. Saunders Co., Philadelphia.)*

the immune system will keep these hypersensitivity reactions under control by decreasing the amount of antibody IgE, IgG, and $T_{dh}$ cells that are produced. That means the levels are never high enough to cause any serious inflammation.

Also, the body can produce "blocking antibodies" of the IgA type that can bind to the allergen in the intestinal tract and inactivate it before it can do any harm. But this balancing act may be thrown off if there is a disease process that allows an increased amount of allergen to enter the body and overwhelm the suppressive control of the immune system.

## Diagnosing Food Allergy

One thing to keep in mind with food allergy is that it can occur in any age pet. The suspicion of food allergy is heightened in puppies or kittens less than one year of age, or in an adult animal that is seven years or older and has never had problems with pruritus before. Between these ages (1-6 years) inhalant allergies (atopy) are the primary causes of non-parasite-related itching. However, since it is not uncommon for individuals to be both food allergic and atopic, age of onset cannot be relied upon to differentiate food allergy from inhalant allergy (atopy).

Before considering food allergy as the cause of the problem, your veterinarian will probably want to do some testing or try medications to make sure that your pet is not suffering from flea bite allergy (much more common than food allergy), mange, bacterial skin infections, or other skin problems that cause pruritus. Skin testing may be needed to determine the presence of inhalant allergies. Many methods have been tried to test for food allergy. Although the intradermal skin test is an effective method for inhalant allergy testing, it has not proven useful for diagnosing food allergy. There are tests available that measure the level of circulating IgE, however it is possible to find high levels of IgE to a specific food and yet not have a reaction to that food.

The test that is considered the most diagnostically useful is the hypoallergenic (restrictive) diet trial.

## The Hypoallergenic Diet Trial

Since we know that food allergy occurs after an individual has been exposed to a certain food, we determine the presence of food allergy by feeding a diet which has ingredients that the individual has never eaten.

### Change the Protein

Since the most common offending allergens are proteins, the first step is to find a diet which has a new protein source. Since beef is the most common protein used in pet foods, and the most common food allergen in the West, we try to avoid it and use instead lamb, rabbit, venison, or legumes such as beans or peas. For years, homemade diets have been used to diagnose food allergy, and some veterinary dermatologists feel that the homemade diet is superior to commercial foods since it theoretically has fewer or no additives.

One important drawback that must be considered with homemade diets is their potential to be nutritionally deficient. They tend to have higher levels of protein and phosphorus and lower levels of calcium, thiamine, and iron than is required for maintaining the adult dog or cat. This could be hazardous for the growing puppy or kitten whose metabolism depends on the continual supply of calcium, vitamins, and minerals that a commercially balanced diet provides. Opinions vary as to whether taurine, an essential amino acid for cats, needs to be supplemented. Some individuals feel that if the homemade diet is used for only two months, the levels of taurine will be adequate for an adult cat for that time period. However, it may be prudent to use a commercial diet for kittens and puppies to avoid causing nutritional deficiencies.

### Test-Feed the Diet

Once a diet is chosen, it is fed exclusively and for a period of time that is felt by the veterinarian to be an adequate test. To help alleviate any problems with diarrhea or constipation that may occur whenever a new diet is fed, it is

# HOMEMADE DIETS

*Homemade diets are not intended for maintenance of adult dogs and cats. They should not be used in immature puppies and kittens.*

## Lamb and Rice Diet:

| | |
|---|---|
| 1 lb. | diced lamb |
| 6 cups | cooked brown rice |
| 4 tsp. | safflower oil |

*Cook rice according to package instructions using purified water. Brown lamb in frying pan or microwave. Combine lamb and all juices with rice. Do not season meat. Yield- 4 lbs. approx.*

Suggested amount to feed:

| Body weight | Amount |
|---|---|
| 5lb | 1/3 lb. |
| 10lb | 1/2 lb. |
| 20lb. | 1 lb. |
| 40lb. | 1 1/2 lb. |
| 60lb. | 2 lb. |
| 80lb. | 2 1/2 lb. |

*The following lamb and rice diet will supply the minimum daily requirements for adult dogs and cats.*

| | |
|---|---|
| 1/4 lb. | lamb |
| 1 cup | cooked rice |
| 1 tsp. | safflower oil |
| 1 1/2 tsp | dicalcium phosphate |
| 1/8 tsp. | potassium chloride |

*Cook rice in pan or microwave. Cook rice following package directions. Mix ingredients. Yield 2/3 lb. Feed same amount that your pet normally eats, adjusting amount to maintain body weight.*

## All-Vegetable Diet:

*1. Vegetable puree [multiple batch]*

*Three undrained #1 cans of:*
*carrots, peas, green beans, tomatoes, and greens (kale, dock, spinach, or mustard).*
*One 10 oz. package of chopped, frozen, broccoli.*

*Boil the broccoli in 2 cups of water until tender. Combine with other vegetables in a large kettle, mix and puree until smooth. Fill 18 one pint plastic containers and freeze.*

*2. Rice [prepare as required]*

*2 1/2 cups rice*
*5 cups water*
*1/2 cup sunflower oil*
*1 tsp salt*

*Mix ingredients, bring to boil, reduce heat and simmer until water is absorbed. Allow to cool.*

*3. Thaw 1 pint of vegetable puree and add to rice, mix thoroughly.*

*4. Feed 1/2 - 3/4 cup per 10 lbs body weight twice daily. Monitor weight weekly. Do not add meat supplements.*

# COMMERCIAL DIETS

Hill's prescription diet d/d

Innovative Veterinary Diets lamb, venison, rabbit, or duck and potato (for dogs).*

Innovative Veterinary Diets lamb, venison, and rabbit and potato (for cats).*

Nature's recipe lamb and rice canned.

Nature's recipe rabbit and rice canned.

Nature's recipe venison and rice canned.

*\* as of this writing, a new product that may not be available in all areas.*

*Ed. note: Both Natural Life's Lamaderm and Precise also make hypoallergenic diets.*

advisable to introduce the new diet gradually over a period of two to three days. For many years, a three-week diet trial was considered adequate to diagnose food allergy. However, because we've learned that the inflammation and pruritus (and so the clinical signs) of food allergy may take a very long time to disappear, the current trend has been to increase that time-period to as long as eight or 10 weeks. Water is the only other item offered, and rawhide chew toys are put away for the duration of the test. Chewable vitamins (especially beef-flavored) are also avoided. Find out if your veterinarian would like you to use a non-flavored supplement. Often your pet may not like the new food or the fact that it is not able to get the treats that it has grown accustomed to.

Warming the new food to enhance the aroma is helpful, and you can alleviate the need for treats a little by keeping some of the food in a separate container in the refrigerator to give out as a treat. This way your pet thinks it is getting something special. The amount to feed varies on the type of diet that your veterinarian selected. Whatever amount you feed it is important to monitor your pets weight weekly to make sure your pet does not lose (or gain!) weight. Some cats may be very finicky, and it may be necessary to try different diets to find the one that the cat likes. It is generally not healthy for a cat (especially an obese one) to go without food for more than two to three days. If this is a problem, call your veterinarian.

If your pet is food allergic, does not have any other conditions causing skin disease or "GI" problems, and the chosen test diet is a good one for your pet, you will notice improvement. If your pet's main problem was pruritus, you may notice less scratching. If the problem was diarrhea, you may see normal bowel movements. The speed with which this recovery occurs varies depending on the individual. It could take as long as eight to 10 weeks. The improvement can be quite dramatic, especially in cats.

### Challenge the Findings

An important step which can aid in determining exactly what your pet is allergic to is to "challenge" your pet with its old food for 10 days and see if signs reappear. If they do, and the signs disappear again after two weeks (or less) back on the hypoallergenic diet, then you can be sure that at least some of your pet's problem was due to a food hypersensitivity. Some pet owners elect to try feeding individual ingredients of the old food, such as beef by itself or corn to see exactly which is the offending food allergen. There is some benefit in knowing what ingredients to avoid when shopping for foods for your pet.

### Maintain the Diet

After food allergy has been determined, the next step is to put your pet on a maintenance diet that your pet can eat indefinitely without harm. If the test diet was a commercial one, you can simply continue to offer it to your pet. If you used a homemade diet, you will probably need to find a commercial diet that contains the same protein and carbohydrate source in a balanced form. Sometimes signs can recur until you find the diet that agrees with your pet. There are some reported cases of pets for which no commercial diet seemed to be adequate for maintenance. If your pet needs to stay on some sort of homemade diet, it will need to be supplemented with adequate calcium, vitamins, minerals, and essential fatty acids to prevent nutritional deficiencies. Speak to your veterinarian or an animal nutritionist.

If your pet did not improve with the diet trial, other possible causes for your pet's problems will need to be addressed.

# Autoimmune Diseases

*By Dr. Alexander Werner, Los Angeles, California*

The immune system is a complex organization of cells and molecules that is specifically designed to distinguish "self" from "non-self." *Self* is defined as substances naturally pertaining to the body, while *non-self* pertains to everything else. The body is under continual attack by an invading world, and the immune system acts as its protecting army. When an invader enters the body, the immune system goes into action — seeking, surrounding, destroying and eliminating these unwanted foreign substances. Called *antigens*, these foreign substances can be infectious agents, proteins or other molecules.

The immune system functions like a well-ordered military, with highly regulated "units" that need to work in close coordination with each other in order to win the battle against antigens. Unfortunately, the immune system doesn't always function at its best. It can "malfunction" in three ways: It may fail to react (immunodeficiency); it may over-react (hypersensitivity); or it may attack *self* instead of *non-self* (auto-immunity).

## Immunodeficiency

Immunodeficiency is simply the lack of an effective immune response. The failure of the body to respond to antigens can be devastating. The current tragedy of AIDS is blamed on a virus which destroys one part of the immune system, thereby weakening one link in the chain and leaving victims with no effective protection against most infections.

### Hypersensitivity

Hypersensitivity is a condition in which the immune system responds excessively against common substances. A common term for hypersensitivity is "allergy." The hypersensitive immune system releases so many chemicals, such as histamine, that the body itself becomes inflamed. Hypersensitivity is discussed in detail in other chapters.

### Autoimmunity

Autoimmunity means "self-destruction." Like an air force that attacks its own cities, the immune system can turn against normal components of the body. It fails to distinguish self from non-self, and attacks body tissues. The specific signs of disease depend on which parts of the body are attacked. This chapter will examine the various dermatological effects that this "friendly fire" can have on our pets.

## The Underlying Causes

Many hypotheses have been offered, but researchers are still unsure about the actual underlying causes of auto-immune disorders. Regardless, there is no doubt that the immune system can go haywire. The *auto-reactive* cell or molecule is one that has been programmed to attack the healthy body tissues. Usually, auto-reactive cells are continually suppressed, preventing an auto-immune disorder. When these mechanisms fail to hold back the auto-reactive cells, trouble begins. The immune system can attack the body in two ways:

•Specialized immune system cells (lymphocytes) may attack the tissue directly.

•Specific molecules (antibodies) may attach to the tissue and begin an inflammatory response.

With either mechanism, the result is the same: The target tissue is damaged or destroyed. A number of auto-immune disorders primarily target, or frequently involve, the skin. (See Table 9.3). As a rule, these skin diseases tend to produce signs around the face and orifice margins (ears, lips, toes, genitalia). Clinical signs are based on which layer or portion of the skin is being attacked.

The skin can be divided into two sections: epidermis and dermis. The *epidermis* is the upper section, which is arranged in distinct layers in a "brick and mortar" fashion — individual cells are the "bricks," and the compound holding them together is the "mortar." The *dermis* is the lower section of the skin. It provides nutrients and support to the epidermis. The dermis is separated from the epidermis by a thin sheet of strong tissue called the *basement membrane*.

Diagnosis of auto-immune skin diseases can be difficult, and almost always requires one or more *biopsies*. Biopsy samples are small pieces of skin tissue that are removed from diseases sites. For the sake of comparison, veterinarians may also take samples of normal skin. These tissue samples are specially preserved, prepared, sliced into sections and examined under a microscope. It is critical that a specially trained veterinary pathologist carefully examine these tissue samples, looking for characteristic changes in the skin as it undergoes the auto-immune process. Biopsies may include special diagnostic tests, such as *immunofluorescent* studies.

# Pemphigus Complex

The four diseases within the *pemphigus complex* share a similar mechanism of destruction: Auto-antibodies ("self" antibodies) adhere to specific parts of the epidermis, and initiate an immune response. The typical response is to dissolve the "mortar" that keeps the cells attached to each other. As the skin falls apart, blisters and ulcers form.

### Pemphigus Foliaceus
Pemphigus foliaceus is the most common disease in the pemphigus complex (see Table 9.3). The breeds most at risk are the Akita, chow chow, dachshund, bearded collie, Newfoundland, Doberman pinscher, and schipperke. In this disease, the auto-antibodies adhere near the skin surface. The resulting blisters are very thin, and they break open almost immediately, producing a crust composed of skin cells and blister fluid. Pemphigus foliaceus usually begins on the face, nose, lips and ears, and may involve the foot pads and groin, but rarely affects the mouth. In severe cases, lesions may be found all over the body. The prognosis is guarded, but medications can control this condition in many animals, keeping them comfortable.

### Pemphigus Erythematosus
Pemphigus erythematosus is a less common, less severe variant of *pemphigus foliaceus*. Lesions are similar, but almost always confined to the face and ears. An ANA test (for explanation, see Systemic Lupus Erythematosus) may be positive. Treatment of pemphigus erythematosus and pemphigus foliaceus is similar, but with a better prognosis in pemphigus erythematosus. Collies and German shepherd dogs may be predisposed to this rare disease.

### Pemphigus Vulgaris
Pemphigus vulgaris is the most severe variant of the pemphigus complex. In

## *Cutaneous Autoimmune Diseases*

| Disease | Common Clinical Signs | Diagnostic Tests | Breed Association |
|---|---|---|---|
| Pemphigus Foliaceus | Face, ear and foot pad crusting | Lesion biopsy | Akita, chow chow, dachshund, schipperke, Doberman pinscher, Newfoundland, bearded collie |
| Pemphigus Erythematosus | Face and ear crusting only | Lesion biopsy; ANA test | Collie, German shepherd |
| Pemphigus Vulgaris | Mouth and orifice ulceration, face ear and body crusting | Lesion biopsy | None |
| Pemphigus Vegetans | Face, ear and body crusting | Lesion biopsy | None |
| Bullous Pemphigoid | Mouth and orifice ulceration; axillae, inguinal, foot pad, toenail crusting and ulceration | Lesion biopsy | Doberman pinscher |
| Systemic Lupus Erythematosus | Variable organ system involvement; hair loss, scaling, ulceration; loss of pigmentation | Lesion biopsy; positive ANA test; organ dysfunction | Collie, German shepherd, Shetland sheepdogs |
| Discoid Lupus Erythematosus | Nasal, muzzle and lip loss of pigment; nasal erosion and bleeding | Lesion biopsy | Germand shepherd, Shetland sheepdog, Siberian husky, collie |
| Cutaneous Lupus Erythematosus | Face and ear hair loss and depigmentation | Lesion biopsy; negative ANA test | None |
| Uveodermatologic Syndrome (VKH) | Nasal, eyelid margin and lip depigmentation; severe eye disease | Lesion biopsy; Eye exam | Akita, Samoyed, Siberian husky |

*Table 8.3*

this disease, the auto-antibodies attach deeper in the skin layers and the destruction produces deep ulcers that usually become infected. The mouth and other body orifices are commonly affected. These animals are quite ill, and their prognosis is grave. No particular breed has been associated with pemphigus vulgaris.

### Pemphigus Vegetans

Pemphigus vegetans is the fourth and rarest variant of the pemphigus complex. Lesions are similar to pemphigus vulgaris, but are usually less severe. The prognosis is guarded. Pemphigus vegetans may represent a "benign" form of pemphigus vulgaris.

## Bullous Pemphigoid

Less common than the four pemphigus complex diseases is *bullous pemphigoid*. It appears most frequently in the Doberman pinscher, but has been seen in other breeds and in mixed-breed dogs. In bullous pemphigoid, the auto-antibody binds between the epidermis and the dermis in the basement membrane, and the blister that forms has a very thick roof. Ulcers commonly develop in the mouth and body orifices (*mucocutaneous junctions*). Lesions may also appear in the *axillary* and *inguinal regions*, foot pads and toenail beds. The disease process is unpredictable: Dogs may be severely ill, or appear quite well apart from their ulcers. The prognosis varies with the severity of the disease.

## Lupus Erythematosus Complex

*Lupus erythematosus* is a disease complex with several variants. In lupus, auto-antibodies are produced against one or more body tissues. Common initiating events include ultraviolet light exposure and administration of some drugs. After the inciting event damages the skin cells, the body perceives the cells as non-self and initiates the immune response in the form of auto-antibodies. In human medicine, the lupus erythematosus complex is subdivided into many separate diseases because prognosis and therapy is different for each variant. In veterinary medicine, this distinction is less clear, and only three diseases have been recognized. These are *systemic lupus erythematosus, cutaneous lupus erythematosus* and *discoid lupus erythematosus*.

### Systemic Lupus Erythematosus

Systemic lupus erythematosus is an uncommon disease that affects more than one body tissue. Skin disease is not usually the most significant symptom of systemic lupus erythematosus. Most signs associated with this disease are varied and can change. Systemic lupus erythematosus has been called "the great imitator" because of its ability to produce such a multitude of signs. Frequently the kidneys, muscle and joints are affected with resultant organ failure. When present, skin lesions are also diverse and include scaling, hair loss, ulceration and loss of pigment. As with other auto-immune diseases, the face and ears are commonly involved. Because of the variability of both clinical signs and laboratory findings, the diagnosis of systemic lupus erythematosus is difficult and relies on several different tests — including tests of organ function, biopsies and a positive antinuclear antibody (ANA) test. The ANA test detects the presence of auto-antibodies against the inside components of the body's cells.

### Discoid Lupus Erythematosus

Discoid lupus erythematosus is the most common skin-related auto-immune disease. It may represent a benign form of systemic lupus erythematosus in which disease is confined to the skin, while other organs are unaffected. Lesions most frequently begin as pigment loss on the nose, and continue with pigment loss on the muzzle and lips. Discoid lupus erythematosus is primarily a cosmetic disease, although severe cases may develop scabs, nasal destruction and recurrent bleeding. Exposure to sunlight increases the severity of this disease. Discoid lupus erythematosus is most frequently seen in collies, German shepherds, Shetland sheepdogs and Siberian huskies. It is frequently referred to as "nasal solar dermatitis," or "collie nose." Diagnosis is made by examining biopsy tissues, and from the absence of disease in other organs. The prognosis is generally excellent, but the disease demands long-term treatment, and relapses are possible.

### Cutaneous Lupus Erythematosus

Cutaneous lupus erythematosus is seen as something of a crossover between discoid and systemic lupus erythematosus. These dogs do not have positive ANA tests, but clinical signs suggest that more often the disease is more aggressive than the relatively benign, facially oriented discoid lupus erythematosus. Prognosis in cutaneous lupus erythematosus is guarded: dogs may remain healthy or their disease may progress into other organs.

# Vogt-Koyanagi-Harada-like Syndrome

A rare disease that affects the pigmented cells in the body, Vogt-Koyanagi-Harada-like syndrome (VKH, or uveodermatologic syndrome) is seen most frequently in Akitas, Samoyeds and Siberian huskies. Skin lesions are striking,

## Therapeutic Agents For Cutaneous Auto-Immune Diseases

| Drug | Trade Name | Side Effects | Recommended Monitoring |
|------|-----------|--------------|------------------------|
| Azathioprine | Imuran | Bone marrow suppression, vomiting, diarrhea, skin rash, depression, hair loss and pancreatitis | Complete blood and platelet counts monthly Not for use in cats |
| Chlorambucil | Leukeran | Bone marrow suppression | Complete blood count and urinalysis monthly |
| Cyclophosphamide | Cytoxan | Sterile hemorrhagic cystitis, vomiting, diarrhea (bloody), hair loss, bone marrow suppression | Complete blood count and urinalysis monthly |
| Cyclosporine | Sandimmune and Cyclosporine A | Vomiting, diarrhea, gum disease, bacterial infections, bone marrow suppression | Periodic drug serum concentration Monthly blood work and urinalysis |
| Glucocorticoids | Prednisone/ Prednisolone and Dexamethasone | Increased thirst, urination, appetite, decreased muscle mass, panting, behavioral changes, vomiting, diarrhea, weight gain, stomach irritation, ulcers | Routine blood work and urine cultures every three months |
| Gold Therapy | Auranofin, Ridaura and Solganol | Severe skin rashes, kidney disease, bone marrow suppression | Blood work and urinalysis weekly for three months, then monthly Use only with corticosteroids |
| Tetracycline and Niacinamide | Tetracycline and Niacinamide* | Loss of appetite, vomiting | Routine blood work every three months |

Table 8.4          *(not to be confused with Niacin)

with complete loss of pigmentation from the normally black lips, nose, and eyelid margins, as well as a whitening of facial hairs. Structures inside the eyes are often the first to be affected, resulting in a sudden onset of inflammation, pain and potential blindness. Diagnosis is made by concurrent eye and skin disease, and is confirmed by biopsy. The prognosis is fair, provided that eye disease can be controlled before blindness occurs.

## Treatment of Autoimmune Disorders

The treatment of auto-immune disorders involves *immunosuppressive* medications which inhibit the body's self-destruction and calm the inflammation. This process requires balancing the suppression of the immune system's destructive forces while attempting to maintain protection against infection.

Constant monitoring for side-effects and secondary infections is critical. There are four basic guidelines that veterinarians follow when devising therapy for auto-immune diseases: combination therapy (using more than one type of drug) may be preferable; the smallest effective dose will result in the least side-effects; pet owners need to be familiar with the expected side-effects; and frequent monitoring for complications is paramount.

The mainstay of immunosuppressive therapy are the glucocorticoids (steroids), which are frequently used to achieve remission. Once in remission, other drugs may be used for continued control. The glucocorticoids cause many side-effects, and that is why they are used sparingly and in combination with other immunosuppressive medications when possible. Other drugs available for treatment of auto-immune disease are selective immunosuppressors — they primarily affect only specific parts of the immune system. When used appropriately, they are safe and can reduce the dosage and side-effects of glucocorticoids. Routine monitoring is crucial for the safety of the animal and cannot be over-emphasized. (Alternative drugs and their names, side-effects and monitoring recommendations are listed in Table 9.4.)

In addition to glucocorticoids and selective immunosuppressors, there are other things that pet owners can do to help reduce the severity of these diseases. These include keeping pets out of the sun, applying sunscreens to exposed areas when outdoors, and — in some instances — giving vitamin E supplementation in the diet.

These extra steps can be very helpful in making sure veterinarian-supervised therapy is going well.

# Contact Allergy and Irritant Contact Dermatitis

*By Dr. Steven A. Melman, Potomac, Maryland*

Typically, when a dog or cat suffers from severe itching (pruritus), the likely cause is an allergic reaction to something the pet has breathed in — the animal kingdom's version of hayfever, what veterinarians call Type I hypersensitivity or inhalant allergy. But that's not always the case. Sometimes, an animal's fits of scratching may be caused by an immune-system reaction to a substance that comes in contact with the pet's skin — what is known as Type 4 contact hypersensitivity, or *contact dermatitis*. A lot of animals suffer similar contact hypersensitivities from things such as laundry detergents, carpet cleaners, soaps, floor waxes, etc. Whereas most animals will be "sensitive" to the irritation of these things, a few people are *excessively* sensitive to a *minute* amount of the offending substance. Such people are considered hypersensitive — suffering from what is called "contact hypersensitivity." Luckily for cats, veterinarians report few cases of felines coming down with a contact dermatitis. But unfortunately for dog owners, contact dermatitis is quite common in canines. However, recent advances in research technology have empowered today's veterinarian with tools that can make proper diagnosis (and subsequent treatment) much more reliable. Nevertheless, making a contact dermatitis diagnosis is not an easy job.

## Making the Diagnosis

Normally, the first step is to make sure the pet is not suffering from an inhalant allergy, especially since the two ailments share so many common symptoms. Other diseases which can commonly cause similar clinical signs must also be eliminated as suspects. This list includes food allergy, scabies (pressure point pruritus), and demodex for feet lesions. Unfortunately, the diagnosis work-up for contact dermatitis is somewhat more difficult, it is also somewhat expensive and may not be readily available to all clinicians. One thing to look for is whether or not more than one pet in the household is suffering from similar symptoms. Because the itching and lesions are caused by a hypersensitivity, it is unlikely that more than one pet in the same household will come down with them.

The only confirmed breed predisposed to contact hypersensitivity is the Danish German shepherd, although other dogs that show high predisposition to allergies in general are the West Highland white terrier, Scottish terrier, golden retriever and the wire-haired fox terrier. It appears that hair can form a protective barrier between the sensitive skin and the offending substance. That may explain why the palms and feet are more commonly affected. Other areas affected include those body sections which come into contact with other surfaces, such as the ventral chest, neck, abdomen and pressure point areas. In some dogs the ear, muzzle and scrotum may be affected. When chew toys or feeding dishes are the offending substances, the canine muzzle will often be the primary location for lesions. The primary clinical sign of contact dermatitis is itching, with redness (erythema), tiny bumps (papules) and occasional small fluid-filled vesicles seen early in the disease process. Chronic signs of skin disease include thickening of the skin, with increased and accentuated lines (lichenification), hyperpigmentation and secondary infection and seborrhea.

### Diagnostic Tests

There are a couple of tests which can help the veterinarian determine that the

## *Causes of Contact Hypersensitivity*

### *Outdoors*
Vegetation, including plants such as *Tradescantia* (wandering Jew) and occasionally grass;
Concrete from the porch, garage or runs;
Cleaning agents used on floor or sidewalk surfaces;
Mulch, which may be contaminated with molds and other chemicals.

### *Indoors*
Insecticides such as pyrethrins employed in flea-kill collars, powders, dips, shampoos and grooming products;
Collars (with or without insecticides);
Bedding;
Carpeting (the offending agent may be the fiber, dye or liner);
Carpet cleaning solutions;
Clothing and other fabrics;
Laundry detergents and softeners;
Flooring, including tile or hardwood;
Floor cleaners, including waxes.

Table 8.5

pet is suffering from a contact dermatitis, and not some other ailment:

- *The European Standard Battery* is a standardized Patch Test that has recently been described as useful in the diagnostic work-ups for dogs. The animal must not be on corticosteroids (no prednisone) for three to six weeks. Generally, the dog should be hospitalized the day before and for 24 hours after the test.

- *The Restriction-Provocation Test* is the best way to confirm the diagnosis. It involves keeping the ailing animal away from potential antigens (the offending substances), and observing very carefully to see whether or not the clinical signs are lessening or even disappearing. Once the dog shows signs of improvement, the offending substance should be re-introduced (either to the environment or directly). All this can take place in the animal clinic, where the pet will be bathed in a hypo-allergenic shampoo and kept in a non-offending environment for 10 to 30 days until the signs abate. Once the animal is re-introduced to an offending substance or environment, the clinical signs will return within 10 days.

## Treatment

The best treatment is to identify the avoiding substance, and avoid it. Hypersensitization has not yet been proven either practical or effective in the treatment of dogs. Occasionally, socks or shirts can be worn by a patient to shield the pet from an offending substance that cannot otherwise be avoided. In the short-term, corticosteroids can be effective. But with time the clinical signs will worsen if the offending substance is not identified and removed. That's why owners must work with their veterinarians in finding that final solution. Unfortunately, if you bring together a group of veterinary dermatologists, the conversation will undoubtedly turn to complaints about lackadaisical owner compliance in the work-up and therapy. So if you love your dog, you'll do what the veterinarian says — for your dog's sake.

## Irritant Contact Dermatitis

Unlike contact hypersensitivity, which is largely an ailment that afflicts individual animals with extremely sensitive immune systems, *irritant contact dermatitis* is something that most animals can suffer from. It results when a pet's skin comes in contact with something such as a harsh chemical or toxic substance. It may even result from a hard physical object. Since the cause-and-effect relationship can be recognized by an observant pet owner, the situation is normally handled adequately at home. Veterinarians only come into the picture when owners cannot figure out what is harming their beloved pets. Clinical signs usually begin suddenly, and they don't normally involve pruritus. More often, the signs are redness, discomfort and pain. Chronic or severe cases may advance into ulcerations and exudation (oozing). What body parts are affected, and the size of the affected skin area, depends in large part on the makeup of the offending substance — while the severity of the ailment is directly tied to the concentration of the material. If it is a liquid that is applied to the body by spray — such as a flea spray — the parts of the body that have been sprayed will be most affected. This brings up an important point: If a substance that causes an irritant reaction is placed on the patient enough times, it may cause the immune system to respond with a contact dermatitis. At some point, further exposure would lead to a full-blown immune-system reaction. This is rarely recognized in dogs, although I have witnessed this happening when pyrethrin flea sprays were used.

As a pet owner, you need to remember there are differences between human and animal skins (see page 54). Those differences can dictate why something which is perfectly fine on human skin will act as an irritant on canine skin. For example, your dog's skin is much thinner, with a more alkaline pH. This means that a shampoo designed for use on human hair may be all wrong for the alkaline pH of the canine skin and coat. If your dog has a serious problem that looks like an acute irritant contact dermatitis, with lesions affecting only the epidermis, the veterinarian will want to perform a biopsy. That will help in making a final diagnosis. Since identification and avoidance of the offending substance are paramount, it is not likely that Patch testing will be necessary. The ailing pet should be bathed in a gentle, hypo-allergenic shampoo such as DermaPet Conditioning Shampoo or Mycodex HA, which will clean and relieve the skin without causing any adverse reactions. Shampoos with medicated substances should be avoided, unless a secondary infection or seborrhea requires their use.

---

## *Causes of Irritant Contact Dermatitis in Dogs*

### *Chemicals*

Soaps, shampoos (benzoyl peroxide, tree oils, betadine, chlorhexidine), detergents, insecticides (especially flea collars), solvents, fertilizer, diesel oil, strong corrosive acids and alkali, petroleum distillates and solvents.

### *Physical Stimuli*

Clippers (particularly No. 40 blades), rough carpets, coarse plants and vegetation (such as thorns or cacti needles).

---

*Table 8.6*

# 9

# ENDOCRINOLOGY

## Overview of Endocrine Abnormalities

*Anthony A. Yu, Auburn, Alabama*

Endocrine skin disorders are often frustrating, in terms of obtaining a clear diagnosis, yet rewarding in terms of response to therapy. For example, hormone disorders generally do not cause itching, yet they are often complicators in dogs that have itchy skin disorders such as allergies, pyodermas and yeast infections. Overdiagnosis of a hormonal disease often results from relying on low baseline (non-stimulated) levels. In this case, a low level may be difficult to assess for various reasons; a test which measures levels obtained from a stimulated organ such as a TSH (thyroid stimulating hormone) test is much more reliable.

Further, depending upon the hormone, the available tests leave a lot to be desired in terms of establishing a clear diagnosis. Thus, while endocrine dermatoses can be one of the most difficult to assess, they can also be one of the most rewarding (next to scabies), in that we are able to elicit a cure—as in the case of Sertoli Cell tumor (via castration)—or control a properly diagnosed dermatopathy such as hypothyroidism with relative ease.

When attempting a diagnosis, the veterinarian must always remember to look at the clinical signs, physical examination findings and test results. That can take some time, as will any ensuing treatment.

It is during treatment that pet owners need to practice the most patience, since handling a hormone imbalance may take time. After all, the veterinarian is attempting to manipulate the narrow confines of a circulating hormone along with complex networks of feedback loops and receptors located throughout the body.

Then again, you may be one of the lucky pet owners whose animals are cured the first time around with one dose of pills. But that's generally the exception, as far as treating hormonal disorders go.

The two most common canine endocrine dermatoses are canine Cushing's syndrome and hypothyroidism. However, I feel that hypothyroidism has been overdiagnosed, and that canine Cushing's syndrome is far more common. Other uncommon disorders include sex hormone imbalances and growth hormone responsive alopecia.

As for felines, what was once thought to be "endocrine alopecia" is now generally recognized as traumatic hair pulling frequently associated with allergic dermatitis. When it comes to glandular problems, cats are generally more fortunate than dogs. That's why the large part of this chapter will focus on dogs, since cats have somewhat fewer outstanding hormonal horror stories.

# Hypothyroidism

One of the most common endocrinopathies in veterinary medicine, but that may be largely a result of veterinary overdiagnoses based on the over-interpretation of baseline thyroxine (T4) concentrations. To complicate matters, the clinical signs of hypothyroidism bear a tremendous resemblance to non-thyroidal illnesses (NTI), which in turn may suppress serum thyroxine levels and lead to misdiagnosis of the disease process.

Veterinary medicine has not yet achieved the diagnostic ability to differentiate between the hypothyroid and euthyroid-sick individuals—an advantage now limited to human medicine. (This is probably because there is no species-specific procedure for evaluating endogenous—naturally made by the body—circulating thyroid stimulating hormone [cTSH] and the recent introduction of unbound, or free, thyroid hormone assays to the veterinary reference laboratories.)

Thyroid hormones are very important. They are closely connected to the growth, development, and function of all organs. If the body fails to synthesize, secrete or use the thyroid hormone, the repercussions are evident internally and externally. The result will be disorders of the reproductive, gastrointestinal, immunologic, cardiovascular, neuromuscular and hematologic systems—all of which are often preceded by dermatologic manifestations. In a very real sense, the skin disorders can provide the alert veterinarian with an early warning bell before more serious and life-threatening problems set in.

Those early warning bells include alopecia (hair loss), which varies from bilaterally symmetrical to localized and asymmetrical. Alopecia is the most common symptom of hypothyroidism, and the one which brings the majority of worried pet owners to the clinic. The hair loss is most prominent along the ventrolateral thorax and abdomen. It is accompanied by hyperpigmentation and a dull, dry coat with guard hairs that epilate (pull out) easily. The coat may lighten in color, become thin and/or develop a texture similar to that of a puppy coat. In later stages, a "rat's tail"—typified by hyperpigmentation and alopecia—may be present.

And despite appropriate therapy, hypothyroid dogs may continue to experience recurrent bacterial pyoderma and otitis externa. Thickened skin—cool to the touch and appearing swollen—is frequently noted in the hypothyroid pet. Afflicted dogs have increased deposits of dermal mucin. This can severely affect the facial region and result in the so-called "tragic expression."

The most common *behavioral* signs noted are lethargy, weakness and a propensity to seek heat. This is because the low circulating levels of thyroid hormone lead to decreased metabolic rates. Naturally, decreases in the heart rate and blood pressure, along with anemia, are ways the body responds to the decreased activity and stimulation.

Commonly, as a result of reduced metabolic activity, the dog gains weight even if it's on a calorie-regulated diet. Dogs with hypothyroidism will suffer from diminished reproductive abilities—in the form of anestrus, irregular cycles, stillborn puppies, lowered sperm levels (azospermia) and decreased libido. The central and peripheral nervous system are also targets of decreased thyroid hormone production and release.

Other signs of hypothyroidism include megaesophagus, bilateral laryngeal paralysis, muscular atrophy, weakness and polyneuropathy, extending to a myxedema coma.

An outward sign that the facial and vestibular nerves have been affected is a droopy eyelid and lip, along with a tilting of the head to one side. A correlation may exist between von Willebrand's disease and hypothyroidism, as depicted by a study where factor VIII and factor VIII-antigen levels paralleled thyroid levels. However, there is not enough data available to assess the exact relationship between hypothyroidism and von Willebrand's disease, or to determine the success of thyroid supplementation alone in reversing this coagulation disorder commonly coexistent in the Doberman pinscher, golden retriever, and miniature schnauzer.

The lack of thyroid hormone in newborn puppies will exacerbate several clinical signs, particularly depressed mental development and dwarfed stature, more commonly known as cretinism.

### Primary hypothyroidism

Primary hypothyroidism, a deficiency in circulating thyroid hormone levels, commonly results from lymphocytic thyroiditis (typified by a damaged thyroid gland). Researchers are still unclear about the cause, but some speculate that prior damage to the thyroid gland and genetic predisposition may be factors.

Idiopathic (cause unknown) atrophy of the thyroid gland is a primary degenerative disorder of the glandular cells with a lack of inflammatory cells. We do not know whether the atrophy is an end-stage form of lymphocytic thyroiditis. However, it accounts for approximately half of all cases of primary hypothyroidism.

Impaired secretion of thyrotropin stimulating hormone (TSH) or thyrotropin-releasing hormone (TRH) is known as *secondary* and *tertiary hypothyroidism*, respectively.

### Secondary hypothyroidism

Secondary hypothyroidism is a dysfunction of the pituitary thyrotrophs. There is insufficient secretion of thyrotropin by the thyrotroph cells of the anterior hypophysis, resulting in thyroid follicular atrophy from the lack of TSH secretion. Suspected causes include congenital malformation of the pituitary gland (an affliction most commonly found in German shepherds), pituitary gland destruction (especially by tumors in older dogs) and suppression of pituitary thyrotroph function secondary to illness, malnutrition or pharmaceuticals.

### Tertiary hypothyroidism

Tertiary hypothyroidism is a dysfunction of the hypothalamus, with insufficient secretion of thyrotropin-releasing hormone by the cells within the paraventricular nucleus of the hypothalamus. As a result, pituitary gland suppression causes thyroid gland atrophy much like secondary hypothyroidism. Potential causes are similar to those of secondary hypothyroidism, including congenital dystrophy, acquired destruction due to neoplasia or hemorrhage, defective TRH molecule, or defective TRH-thyrotroph receptor interaction.

External factors play an important role when evaluating thyroid hormone levels. Clinical signs of hypothyroidism are similar regardless of the location of the lesion. However, dogs with secondary or tertiary hypothyroidism may also have clinical signs which suggest impaired secretion of other pituitary or hypothalamic hormones.

Diagnosis of *adult onset hypothyroidism* is based on an all-encompassing evaluation of the patient. Clinical signs, history and physical exam findings aid tremendously in this goal. Veterinarians take into special consideration the role played by age and breed, since hypothyroidism most commonly develops in middle-aged, medium- to large-breed dogs. The onset of clinical signs occurs at approximately 6 years of age. Great Danes, Doberman pinschers, shar-peis, golden retrievers, Irish setters, boxers and miniature schnauzers seem over-represented in the diagnosis of hypothyroidism. This suggests these breeds are genetically predisposed. The animal's sex does not seem to play a role.

Owners often bring in their pets with complaints of abnormal behavior, including the animal's sudden desire for heat, as well as weight gain in the face of a normal caloric intake, lethargy and weakness. Physical examination then reveals consistent dermatologic lesions, a decreased heart rate and decreased rectal temperature.

(For the veterinarian, evidence to support a positive diagnosis on routine screening tests includes normocytic/normochromic anemia, along with elevated cholesterol, triglyceride, or creatine phosphokinase levels. A urinalysis may reveal an increased white blood cell count secondary to a bacterial cystitis. Bleeding times may be prolonged, as shown by increases in times for activated clotting and partial thromboplastin. Abnormal heart rhythms show up in an electrocardiographic examination, characterized by a slow heart rate with decreased R-wave amplitudes and inverted T-waves. Thus, several routine evaluations may provide insight into a potentially life-threatening endocrinopathy.)

Specific diagnostic measures are needed to conclusively prove hypothyroidism. In human medicine, most hypothyroid cases are diagnosed by measuring free thyroxine (FT4) and circulating thyroid stimulating hormone. Veterinary medicine still lacks a cTSH assay for dogs, cats or horses, because this test is species-specific. Thus, veterinarians acquire a better understanding of the available surveys by relying upon routine screening and stimulation tests.

Physiological considerations arise when performing thyroid evaluations. Young puppies naturally have 2-5 times elevated basal thyroid levels; these decrease to within normal reference limits by 4-5 months of age. The more mature dog often shows decreased baseline and post-stimulation levels.

*Nonthyroidal illnesses comprise the second most common cause of falsely-altered thyroid levels.* Conditions such as chronic renal failure, adrenal gland disease, diabetes mellitus, liver disease and other chronic skin conditions can result in decreased serum baseline thyroid levels. This condition is often termed *euthyroid sick syndrome*; that is, the thyroid is still functional but the body has decreased the production of this hormone in response to the decreased activity experienced during illness. The severity of illness correlates directly with the severity of suppression of serum T4 concentration.

The last but most common cause of falsely altered thyroid hormone levels is the influence of various drugs: in particular, glucocorticoids, phenylbutazone, anticonvulsants, anesthetics, long-term sulfonamide treatment, and radiocontrast dyes. These thyroid gland changes can be reversed with subsequent removal of the inciting agent. The veterinarian must consider these factors when attempting to interpret thyroid hormone laboratory values. Also, (s)he must look at pertinent findings from historical and physical evaluation as well as clinical pathology, and bring a high index of suspicion to his/her evaluation.

## Tests

Specific diagnostic serum tests available include a TSH or TRH stimulation test; measurement of baseline T4, triiodothyronine (T3), free T4 (FT4), free T3 (FT3) and reverse T3 (rT3); and autoantibodies to thyroglobulin (aaTG), T3 (aaT3) and T4 (aaT4). Quite routinely, baseline total T4 levels should be performed. This hormone is the main *secretory* product of the thyroid gland. Serum T4 displays normal fluctuations in basal thyroid hormone concentrations. *Hypothyroid dogs can have serum thyroxine concentration within the resting range of normal dogs.*

Serum T4 measurements are a useful, inexpensive means to evaluate the thyroid status of an individual. The procedure involves a single blood sample and can be processed by most reference laboratories by radioimmunoassays (RIA). Interpretation of baseline T4 values is straightforward, but becomes ambivalent when nonthyroidal illnesses or extraneous factors affect the results of this test.

Thus, a dog with a low T4 (<10 nmol/l, where normal = 20-55 nmol/l), but no concurrent illness or drug administration, can be diagnosed as hypothyroid, if a physical exam produces findings consistent with hypothyroidism. Repeating T4 on three occasions with similar or declining values will support such a diagnosis.

Serum T4 is a useful tool in veterinary medicine, but does not provide high specificity and sensitivity. It therefore must be interpreted cautiously.

The measurement of T3 is often performed needlessly. T3 is a minor product of the thyroid gland; however, it is the major hormone produced at the target tissues. The poor diagnostic ability of serum T3 concentration to discern hypothyroidism may stem partially from a predominance of T4 secretion by the normal thyroid gland, the primary intracellular location of T3, and from the increased thyroidal secretion of T3, with progressive loss of thyroid gland function.

The concept of a defect in the conversion of T4 to T3 has, as of this publication, not been substantiated in veterinary medicine. Elevated levels of T3 are associated with the production of aaT3, which is a rare condition affecting only one percent of the canine population. Also, serum T3 levels are equally influenced by extraneous factors, as are T4 levels. Therefore, routine processing of T3 is invalid in the diagnostic approach to hypothyroidism.

Recently, equilibrium dialysis, a more sensitive and specific (but time-consuming) test, was developed to evaluate FT4. This method provides no additional information on thyroid gland function beyond what is gained by measuring serum T4 concentration.

Other parameters that have been investigated include measurement of reverse T3 (rT3) and thyroid autoantibodies to thyroglobulin (aaTG), T3 (aaT3) and T4 (aaT4). Reverse T3 is supposed to increase in the euthyroid sick individual. Unfortunately, there is little evidence that rT3 helps to distinguish between hypothyroidism and nonthyroidal suppression of T3 and T4. Thyroid autoantibodies are produced as part of the immune mediated lymphoid thyroiditis complex. They often help in early detection and are found even when normal circulating levels of T3 and T4 are present. However, they generally are associated with unusual T4 or T3 values. Circulating thyroid hormone antibodies may interfere with RIA techniques, producing spurious numbers that are not reliable. The type of interference depends on the separation system used in the RIA. Interpreting auto-antibody levels is complex, since even normal dogs display some detectable level of aaTG, while production of aaT3 and aaT4 production is noted so infrequently.

Thyroid scans with intravenously administered radioactive labeled iodide have been used recently to investigate the etiology of sulfonamide-induced decreased serum thyroxine levels.

## TSH Stimulation

Many factors can influence the value of a single thyroid hormone evaluation—with spurious results. To minimize the influence of these factors, experts advocate the TSH stimulation test as the gold standard for diagnosing primary hypothyroidism in the cat, dog and horse. It indicates the functional reserve capacity expressed by the magnitude of response.

Pre- and post-stimulation samples are compared to the normal reference range. A hypothyroid pet will lack a response or show minimal elevations from the baseline value. Most often, the difference in response is easily distinguishable from the euthyroid animals. Borderline responses (i.e., low to low normal pre-TSH value; some increase of T4 in response to TSH) may coincide with nonthyroidal illness, treatment with certain drugs, secondary hypothyroidism, or possibly early stage primary hypothyroidism. The response should be diminished in a subsequent test if the animal is developing primary hypothyroidism.

Unfortunately, the source of TSH used for testing is sparse and costly. This—along with the fact that the results may still be equivocal, especially with nonthyroidal illnesses—makes hypothyroidism difficult to diagnose. *Despite some of these faults, the TSH stimulation test is the most reliable diagnostic test available* to differentiate a borderline T4 value in veterinary medicine until a canine cTSH assay is developed.

Unfortunately, the body's response to exogenously administered TSH does not reflect the function of the hypophysis or hypothalamus. The dose of TSH used in canine and feline thyroid function testing is, undoubtedly, much greater than the quantity of endogenously produced TSH in the pituitary gland. In addition, thyroxine response to TRH stimulation is less than the response to TSH stimulation. This suggests that the TSH stimulation test could be considered a pharmacologic (drug-induced) thyroid function test, rather than a physiologic thyroid function test.

Diagnosis of endocrine dysfunction by stimulation testing is an attempt to evaluate the endocrine regulatory hierarchy. Thus, physiologic testing is more desirable than pharmacologic endocrine function testing. The TRH stimulation test is more a physiologic (hence, more sensitive) thyroid function test than TSH stimulation test, because endogenous production of TSH by the pituitary gland is necessary for normal serum thyroxine response to TRH.

## Treatment

Once a diagnosis has been established, treatment of any concurrent diseases such as bacterial pyodermas, demodicosis, *Malassezia pachydermatis* infection, and seborrhea is recommended. Any residual concurrent diseases may alter the response to thyroid supplementation. The most common dosage regimen used is 0.1 mg/lb once to twice daily. Other recommendations include 0.5 mg/M$^2$ once to twice daily.

Depending on response to therapy, twice-daily medication is preferred. Available products include Synthroid, Soloxine, and Thyro-Tabs. Quite often, in more mature animals with heart conditions, a once-daily regimen followed by an increase to twice daily on a gradual basis will provide satisfactory results without compromising the patient.

It is necessary to monitor the pet on a regular basis due to the dynamic changes that are occurring with respect to body weight and activity level. Within days, the pet's attitude will improve, showing increased alertness and responsiveness, and within 12 weeks the coat should return to normal.

A six-hour post-pill T4 level should be obtained four to six weeks after the initiation of therapy. If low values are obtained and improvement is negligible, the veterinarian may have to reconsider the administration or dosage, bioavailability of the brand of synthetic thyroxine, and possibly another cause of the skin condition. Increasing the dosage or switching to a different brand may provide a better response to therapy.

Re-checking post-pill levels should be continued until a high normal value (45-60 nmol/l) is obtained. Thereafter, sampling every six to 12 months will allow fine adjustments to be made throughout the patient's life.

In summary, hypothyroidism is often misdiagnosed due to overinterpretation of laboratory results. The future holds great prospects for a canine cTSH and further availability of the equilibrium dialysis method of fT4 measurement, which would help in obtaining an accurate diagnosis. Until then, veterinarians must continue to collect historical, clinical and laboratory findings, and scrupulously strive toward a proper diagnosis.

# Sex Hormone Imbalances In The Dog

Sex hormone imbalances are rare. Canine Cushing's Syndrome and hypothyroidism are the most common endocrinopathies diagnosed in the dog, and should be ruled out before pointing the finger at an imbalance of sex hormones as the culprit in a bilateral symmetrical alopecia.

There are five basic conditions to consider:

1) Ovarian imbalance type I;

2) Ovarian imbalance type II;

3) Castration responsive dermatosis;

4) Sex hormone producing testicular tumors; and

5) Testosterone responsive alopecia.

Keep in mind that most of these cases have a bilateral symmetrical alopecia distributed largely over the ventrum, and beginning in the genital region.

Of course, gender will dictate which condition the veterinarian should focus on.

### Ovarian Imbalances

These occur in bitches and are associated with both excessive production (Ovarian imbalance type I) or decreased levels of estrogen (Ovarian imbalance type II). Once again, these are relatively rare conditions. They are characterized by bilateral symmetric alopecia, which begins in the genital region and spreads forward to the ventrum, flank and neck. Subtle differences exist between the two disorders.

Ovarian type I imbalances are associated with the production of excess estradiol, testosterone or progesterone from the ovaries. Naturally, it follows that these conditions are commonly associated with intact female dogs. However, given the availability of estrogens to treat of urinary incontinence and mismating, and the possibility that the dog has accidentally consumed human birth control pills, one must focus on an accurate history to rule out an exogenous source of hormones.

Ovarian imbalance type I, also known as hyperestrogenism, has often been seen in middle- to older-aged intact female dogs with cystic ovaries or functional ovarian tumors. The bilateral, symmetric alopecia may parallel heat cycles, pregnancies or pseudopregnancies, before becoming a year-round problem. Typically, this means other skin changes, such as hyperpigmentation, ceruminous (waxy) otitis externa, seborrhea and pyoderma with associated pruritus. Gynecomastia (large breasts, nipples, clitoris and vulvar enlargement) abnormal heat cycles and recurrent pseudopregnancies will often be noted by breeders.

Diagnosis can be supported by several testing procedures. However, ovariohysterectomy is the method of choice. Not only does it offer a cure—if indeed we are dealing with an excess production of estrogen—but it also will prevent any further medical complications such as pyometra, cystic endometrial hyperplasia, or neoplasia associated with the reproductive tract.

But if the bitch is supposed to continue breeding, then every effort should be made to document an abnormal balance of estrogen. Diagnostic tests would show a predominance of squamous epithelial cells on vaginal smears; evidence of bone marrow suppression such as thrombocytopenia (low platelets), anemia (low red blood cells) and leukopenia (low white blood cells) on a complete blood count; and elevated serum sex hormone levels (estradiol, testosterone, progesterone). The tests would also include visualization of enlarged cysts or tumors on the ovaries on physical exam, by ultrasound or X-ray examination, and skin biopsies.

Samples for sex hormone evaluation offer the best results if taken during diestrus. Also, recent investigations have provided more meaningful results with stimulation tests using gonadotropic releasing hormone (GnRH). However, the cost of analysis of stimulation test samples makes it prohibitive for routine use. Ovariohysterectomy (spaying), with hair regrowth in three to six months, is the most economical method of differentiating an endocrine alopecia attributable to ovarian imbalance type I.

For completeness, the ovaries and uterus should be submitted for biopsy evaluation to verify the absence of malignancy.

Ovarian imbalance type II, or hypoestrogenism, occurs most frequently in dogs spayed at a young age (prior to puberty). The cause is unknown. This extremely uncommon condition also results in a bilaterally symmetric alopecia involving the genital, flank, ventrum and thigh regions, as well as the pinnae.

Ovarian imbalance type II is typified by immature development of the vulva and nipples, lack of hyperpigmentation, and possibly urinary incontinence. Breeds most commonly affected include the dachshund and the boxer.

Diagnosis is difficult and is based on response to estrogen supplementation with diethylstilbestrol in four-week cycles until hair regrowth is noted in approximately eight to 12 weeks. Thereafter, a maintenance schedule of once to twice weekly administration of diethylstilbestrol is recommended.

Side-effects of diethylstilbestrol include anemia, thrombocytopenia and leukopenia. Therefore, routine monitoring of complete blood counts by your veterinarian is strongly encouraged. Further evaluation toward a diagnosis may include baseline and/or post-stimulation evaluation of sex hormones, along with a skin biopsy. Unfortunately, results from the biopsy are often equivocal, with characteristics similar to that of ovarian imbalance type II.

Some extremely rare sex hormone imbalances occur in the female dog. These include ovarian imbalance type II in an intact bitch, which can be treated with follicle stimulating hormone; hyperandrogenism, typified by perianal adenomas, leg-lifting and mounting behaviors, as a result of excess male hormones (e.g., testosterone) secreted by the adrenal cortex; and telogen defluxion occurring six to eight weeks after whelping due to dramatic changes in hormone levels, particularly a drop in circulating estrogen levels.

### Castration-responsive dermatosis.

This is a bilaterally symmetric alopecia and hyperpigmentation. It involves the trunk and neck, sparing the distal extremities. Quite often there is a puppy coat, due to a lack of mature guard hairs with discoloration of dark hair coats turning to a reddish bronze. The condition affects intact, sexually mature male dogs with normal, descended testes. Keeshonds, Siberian huskies, Pomeranians, chow chows, miniature poodles and Alaskan malamutes are at higher risk.

The cause is unknown, although it may be related to an imbalance of gonadal hormones. Resolution of clinical signs is often achieved by castration. Hair regrowth is expected within six months.

Pre-castration diagnosis is difficult, but is sometimes supported by a biopsy of the skin with evidence of so-called "flame follicles," and abnormalities in pre- and/or post-stimulation serum sex hormone evaluation. Decreased response of growth hormone to a xylazine stimulation test has been reported historically with this condition. Unfortunately, to date, no validated canine growth hormone assays exist.

### Testicular Neoplasias

These have been associated with sex hormone-related alopecia, the most common being the Sertoli cell tumor. This tumor frequently develops in older male dogs that have retained testicles. Boxers, weimaraners, German shepherds, Cairn terriers, Pekingeses, collies and Shetland sheepdogs are at higher risk.

Sertoli cell tumors tend to be functional estrogen-producing tumors that cause male feminizing signs such as gynecomastia and behavioral abnormalities. They also cause a bilaterally symmetric alopecia similar to that of Ovarian imbalance type I; that is, a distribution of hair loss involving the flanks and ventrum with evidence of decreased skin thickness and similar histopathological appearance of skin biopsies. A key feature is the presence of a linear dermatosis on the ventral surface of the prepuce. Hyperpigmentation is mainly observed in those male dogs exhibiting signs of feminization. The treatment of choice is castration, with submission of the testicles for histopathologic evaluation.

A presurgical work-up is warranted to screen for evidence of thrombocytopenia and anemia. Abdominal X-rays and ultrasonography may reveal prostatomegaly, an abdominal mass, sublumbar lymph node enlargement or metastasis. Interestingly, a specific syndrome in male miniature schnauzers constitutes Sertoli cell tumors, feminization, male pseudohermaphroditism and cryptorchidism.

### Testosterone Responsive Alopecia

This final sex hormone imbalance is the rarest of those mentioned in this chapter. It is seen in middle-aged male dogs castrated early in life or in older male dogs that may be castrated, are cryptorchid, have atrophied testicles, or have testicular neoplasia.

Clinical signs include a bilaterally symmetric alopecia with a dull, dry coat and thin skin. A diagnosis can be supported by consistently low testosterone levels, and skin biopsy findings consistent with an endocrinopathy. To treat this, a dog should be given methyltestosterone orally. Once the dog has responded to therapy, doses should be tapered to a maintenance regimen.

Adverse effects of therapy may include liver enzyme elevation and/or behavioral modification toward aggression.

## Feline Problems Are Few

There are very few feline endocrine dermatoses. One condition typically seen in intact males is called "stud tail" or tail gland hyperplasia. These cats typically have large amounts of grease, scale and crusts on the dorsal surface of the lower third of the tail. The cause is unknown, and the affected cats respond not to castration, but to the antiandrogenic effects of progestational compounds. Side-effects of prolonged megesterol acetate (Ovaban) include diabetes mellitus, fibroadenomatous mammary gland hyperplasia, cutaneous atrophy and alopecia.

In both feline and canine veterinary dermatology, it is extremely important to exclude the more common causes of alopecia before undertaking the dubious task of documenting a sex hormone-related dermatosis.

Common differentials for a non-pruritic alopecia should include demodicosis, ringworm, hypothyroidism, hyperadrenocorticism, sex hormone dermatosis, growth hormone-responsive alopecia and idiopathic follicular dysplasia. In any case, a diagnostic challenge awaits.

# Growth Hormone Imbalances in the Dog

Growth hormone deficiency is a rare syndrome that is difficult to diagnose and treat. It appears in two different forms, depending upon the age of onset. Growth hormone excess causes acromegaly. First, we will try to understand what growth hormone is.

The release of growth hormone is stimulated by numerous factors—including growth hormone-releasing factor, dopamine, alpha-adrenergic agonists, glucagon, vasopressin and estrogens. Somatostatin—which originates from the hypothalamus, the gastrointestinal tract, and the pancreas—is carried to the anterior pituitary gland, where it inhibits the production of growth hormone, also called somatotropin. The exact role of growth hormone in the skin is not known.

Growth hormone enhances protein synthesis and fat utilization, both directly and by indirect stimulation of mediators, such as somatomedins or insulin-like growth factors, produced in the liver and possibly other tissues. Clinical signs may be a result of excess production or lack thereof.

In the case of growth hormone insufficiency in puppies, the development of a cystic Rathke's pouch is a result of an inherited autosomally recessive condition. The clinical signs of this deficiency are dwarfism, retention of a puppy coat, and development of a bilateral symmetrical alopecia. The breed most commonly affected is the German shepherd.

Because puppies are born "normal," owners will notice nothing wrong for several months, then realize that some dogs have not kept pace with their rapidly-growing littermates. Some of these pituitary dwarfs will also be hypothyroid and Addisonian, since the pituitary gland has produced inadequate levels of TSH and/or ACTH.

Hyposomatotropism in the mature dog has been referred to as growth hormone-responsive dermatosis, pseudo-Cushing's syndrome, and adult onset growth hormone deficiency. Clinical signs appear after one year of age, when the dogs are already of normal stature and size. Given the propensity of the condition in Pomeranians, keeshonds, miniature poodles, American water spaniels and chow chows, this disorder may also be hereditary.

Clinical signs include a loss of primary hairs with retention of secondary hairs to alopecia, and hyperpigmentation of the neck and trunk sparing the face and extremities. The skin on these dogs is thin, as with canine Cushing's syndrome, making it difficult to diagnosis this condition.

Diagnosis is primarily based on signalment, history, physical examination, elimination of other causes, and biopsy for histopathological evaluation.

Unfortunately, there is no commercially available validated canine growth hormone assay. Thus, a diagnosis means discriminating between canine Cushing's syndrome, hypothyroidism, and sex hormone imbalances (in particular testosterone responsive alopecia). Once again, it must be emphasized that diagnostic tests to sufficiently exclude canine Cushing's Syndrome and hypothyroidism—the most frequently encountered endocrine disorders affecting the skin—should be included in any evaluation of a growth hormone-responsive alopecia.

Biopsy findings which suggest growth hormone responsive alopecia include a thin dermis with decreased amounts of dermal elastin fibers.

Treatment consists of subcutaneous injections of porcine and bovine growth hormone every 10 days. Human growth hormone may have some efficacy at

0.15 IU/kg administered subcutaneously twice weekly. Response is usually seen within eight to 12 weeks and remains in remission for six to 24 months. However, these products are produced only in limited quantity, and human medical applications get preference.

As well, growth hormone can lead to diabetes mellitus if serum glucose levels are not monitored consistently. Some Pomeranians also develop Cushing's syndrome.

A condition of excess production of growth hormone—referred to as *acromegaly*—is depicted by enlargement of most body organs, and a thickened, myxedematous dermis. Also, most of these dogs exhibit widened interdigital and interdental spaces, and inspiratory stridor due to an elongated soft palate.

Once again, diagnostics are limited because a validated growth hormone assay is not available. However, most affected dogs have elevated serum glucose levels. This, along with the physical exam findings and biopsy results, strongly suggests acromegaly.

Growth hormone-related dermatoses take on several appearances. With the lack of a validated analyses for canine growth hormone, a diagnosis of these conditions is based largely upon history, physical examination findings, and exclusion of other dermatoses.

# Cushing's Syndrome (Hyperadrenocorticism)

*by Dr. Thomas A. Janik, Chicago, Illinois*

At first glance, Cushing's Syndrome could be easily overlooked in the search to figure out why the canine patient on the examination table is suffering from hair loss, excessive acne, dry skin, hyperpigmentation, obesity, calcium deposits in the skin and other symptoms that are common to numerous dermatological ailments. But these clinical signs of Cushing's Syndrome (also called *hyperadrenocorticism*) include some other unique symptoms, such as excessive thirst, urination and panting, along with a distended belly. It is these last few symptoms that, in conjunction with some of the above, are valuable to the veterinarian, alerting the professional to the possibility of hyperadrenocorticism.

Before we get into a discussion on how to treat this disease, it would be wise to look at the origins of Cushing's Syndrome, an ailment which is much more common in dogs than cats. Those breeds more likely to be affected are miniature poodles, dachshunds and Boston terriers. Gender has nothing to do with it, although the average age of onset has been estimated at eight years.

As the name hyperadrenocorticism implies, this disease is a result of overproductive adrenal glands, which secrete abnormally high levels of glucocorticoids. The adrenal glands, which are located near the kidneys, are divided into two sections (cortex and medulla), each with distinctly different functions. Normally, it is the adrenal cortex which secrets cortisol in response to a hormone (ACTH — adrenal corticotropic hormone) which comes from the pituitary gland (a small structure attached to the bottom of the brain). Sometimes, tiny tumors can form in the pituitary gland, which leads it to overproduce the ACTH hormone. With all that hormone floating around, the adrenal cortex kicks into action and secretes too much cortisol. This malady is known as "pituitary dependent hyperadrenocorticism," or PDH. Another possible, but less common, monkey wrench in the system can be the growth of tumors within the adrenal cortex. This also leads the adrenal glands to produce too much cortisol. And unfortunately for dogs, excessive amounts of cortisol lead directly to the clinical signs of hyperadrenocorticism.

But the origins of Cushing's Syndrome are not limited solely to such internal (endogenous) problems. Cushing's Syndrome can also result from outside influences (exogenous causes), or as a side effect of medically administered glucocorticoids used to treat other illnesses (an iatrogenic cause). The first challenge, however, is making sure the dog or cat is actually suffering from hyperadrenocorticism. Of course, the initial step in this direction is recognizing the clinical signs.

## The Tell-Tale Signs

Pets suffering from "glucocorticoid excess" will suffer from higher blood glucose levels (gluconeogenesis) and increased free-water clearance by the kidneys, as well as anti-inflammatory effects, immunosuppression, and tissue deposition and loss (calcium mobilization). The systemic imbalances will show themselves outwardly as:

- Increased thirst (polydipsia) and urination (polyuria);

- Distended belly (pendulous abdomen);

- Muscle weakness and atrophy;

- Obesity; and

- Increased panting.

The effects on the skin will include:

- Bilateral symmetrical hair loss (alopecia);

- Comedones (pimples or blackheads);

- Calcium deposits in the skin (calcinosis cutis);

- Hyperpigmentation;

- Thin, dry skin which can sometimes appear wrinkled or have an increased elasticity.

On top of that, the animal may experience immunosuppression, decreasing the body's ability to fight infection. The true tell-tale signs of this disease are the polyuria, polydipsia, alopecia and pendulous abdomen.

## Treating the Endogenous Ailment

Once an alarm has been set off, the veterinarian will want to run an array of simple tests on the dog to confirm that the problem really is Cushing's Syndrome. This means putting the animal through a CBC (complete blood count), urinalysis and blood chemistry profile. The veterinarian will be looking for a change in the serum alkaline phosphatase (SAP) level, a liver enzyme. But because this enzyme has more than one source, the veterinarian will have to be sure to determine whether or not the SAP level is steroid-induced. A definitive diagnosis of Cushing's Syndrome requires adrenal function testing. Owners should not be upset if their pets must be hospitalized for a day while undergoing a series of tests. Some of the basic tests that may be used to obtain a final diagnosis include the following:

- ACTH stimulation test (which measures a baseline and one- to two-hour plasma cortisol);

- Low-dose and/or high-dose dexamethasone suppression test (if a low dose of dexamethasone fails to suppress the plasma cortisol, this confirms the presence of Cushing's Syndrome. Then a high-dose dexamethasone suppression test will differentiate a pituitary dependent cause from an adrenal tumor);

- Urine cortisol;

- Plasma ACTH (this is a difficult test to perform and transport — although ideally the best — since it cannot be stored in glass and must be frozen immediately).

What the veterinarian is trying to do with these tests is to identify hyperadrenocorticism and figure out whether or not the dog has tumors of the adrenal gland or of the pituitary gland. The medical professional *must* know this so she can decide what method of treatment to follow. Treatment can be surgical (adrenalectomy) for adrenal tumors, or medical (using the drugs Mitotane "Lysodren" or ketoconazole "Nizoral") for pituitary dependant, or simply withholding all cortisone products (as in the case of iatrogenic Cushing's). If the latter route is followed, Lysodren can be administered orally on a daily basis for between seven and 10 days. Maintenance therapy is then given once or twice weekly, depending on the responses according to ACTH stimulation testing.

Lysodren selectively kills adrenal cortex cells, which can result in just the opposite of Cushing's Syndrome — Addison's Disease. Patients undergoing this alternative drug therapy may show signs of weakness, poor appetite, vomiting and diarrhea.

While receiving Lysodren, dogs may also take oral dosages of ketoconazole twice daily, the effects of which are also monitored on the ACTH stimulation test. The side-effects of this drug can include poor appetite and vomiting. Maintenance therapy dosages are also twice-daily. Both of these drugs are relatively expensive. Medical treatment is ongoing, and not without risks. Careful management and monitoring of progress through regularly scheduled office visits and testing is required.

## Dealing With Corticosteroids

As mentioned earlier, sometimes drugs used to treat other illnesses can lead to the same symptoms of Cushing's Syndrome. Such is the Yin-and-Yang of corticosteroids and related medications which bring relief on one hand, and unwanted side-effects on the other. We are dealing with a group of drugs known as corticoids, glucorcorticoids, corticosteroids (there are other types of steroids), and various cortisone products used to treat a variety of conditions. Unfortunately, the negative side-effects show themselves shortly after use, and they're long-lasting in duration. Since 1949, these commercial preparations have been available, and have since become an important therapeutic tool for veterinarians and physicians alike. They come in many forms: tablets and liquids taken orally; injectable forms given IM, IV or intralesionally; and creams, ointments and solutions for topical use on the skin and in the eyes and ears. All cortisone products — such as the commonly used prednisolone, prednisone, Azium (dexamethasone), Vetalog (triamcinolone) and Depo-Medrol — are modifications of the same basic molecular structure.

Steroids have a great deal of merit in the treatment of a variety of conditions such as head and brain trauma, vestibular disease, disc disease, various eye problems, post-surgical management, immune-medicated diseases and neoplastic diseases. By far, however, it is the skin diseases which are most often treated with this class of drugs. That's because the cortisones give prompt relief for itchy animals. Primarily, these drugs offer anti-inflammatory benefits, thereby reversing those chemical reactions that cause itchiness and hair loss. But they do not correct the root cause of all this discomfort. Sooner or later, the itchiness and hair loss will return — a sign that there is a long road to travel in the search for the primary illness.

Which is not to say that there is no place for steroid use. On the contrary, there are many skin diseases which require and benefit from the long-term use of steroids. And once a final definitive diagnosis has been made, there should be no hesitation over the long-term use of steroids. However, if a veterinarian sees the side-effects beginning shortly after the start of corticosteroid therapy, but makes no attempt at making a further diagnosis or doesn't try any alternative treatment methods, the medical professional is being negligent.

Corticosteroids can affect nearly every cell in the body, causing a wide array of systemic problems:

- •Skin: atrophy, thinning, infection and possible calcium deposition;

- •Skeletal muscle: weakness and atrophy;

- •Central nervous system: euphoria, depression and other behavioral changes;

- •Liver: steroid hepatopathy, increased liver enzymes (serum alkaline phosphatase), increased glucose formation;

- •Kidneys: increased extracellular fluid volume (bloating), increased resorption of water, sodium and chloride (urination);

- •Bone: acceleration of bone resorption (osteoporosis);

- •Hematopoietic (blood system): immuno-suppression, increase in neutrophils, decrease in eosinophils and lymphocytes.

These systemic problems lead to the common side-effects of excessive thirst and urination, lowered resistance to infection, obesity and panting — all of which in turn lead to numerous clinical complications, including iatrogenic hyperadrenocorticism (Cushing's Syndrome). Given the consequences of steroid use, it is the veterinarian's responsibility to see a proper diagnosis. This includes seeking a second opinion, or referring the case to a qualified dermatologist.

# *Pediatric, Congenital & Genetic Disorders*

| *Name of Condition* | *Defect in* | *Animals at Risk* |
|---|---|---|
| Cutaneous asthenia | collagen bundles | dogs & cats |
| Aplasia cutis | skin does not develop | dogs & cats |
| Acanthosis nigricans | melanin pigment | dachshund |
| Familial canine dermatomyositis | inflammed skin & muscle | collie, Shetland sheepdog |
| Acral mutilation syndrome | nerves to feet | German shorthaired pointer, English pointer |
| Acrodermatitis dermoid sinus | zinc absorption, neural tube formation | bull terrier, Rhodesian ridgeback, shih-tzu, boxer |
| Chediak-Higashi syndrome | melanin granule | Persian (smoke color) |
| Color-mutant alopecia | hair production, melanin formation | blue dogs; Doberman pinscher, dachshund, chow-chow, standard poodle, great Dane, Italian greyhound, whippet |
| Feline alopecia universalis | hair formation | Sphinx cat, Canadian hairless cat |
| Feline hypotrichosis | hair formation | Devon rex cat |
| Canine alopecic breeds | hair formation | Mexican hairless, Chihuahua, Abyssianian dog, African sand dog, Turkish naked dog, Peruvian hairless dog, xoloitzcuintl |
| Congenital alopecia | hair formation | Cocker spaniel, Belgian shepherd, beagle, whippet, bichon frise, bassett hound |
| Pattern baldness | hair formation | Yorkshire terriers |
| Melanoderma, alopecia of yorkshire terrier | hair formation | Yorkshire terriers |
| Lymphedema | lymph system | English bulldog, German shepherd, borzoi, Belgian Tervuren, Labrador retriever, great Dane, poodle |
| Tyrosinemia | tyrosine metabolism | German shepherd |
| Collagen disorder of footpads of German shepherd | defect unknown | German shepherd |
| Digital hyperkeratosis of Irish terriers | defect unknown | Irish terrier |
| Juvenile cellulitis | pustules | All dogs |
| Infantile pustular dermatosis | pustules | All dogs |

*Table 10.1*

# 10

# PEDIATRIC, CONGENITAL & HEREDITARY DISEASES

## Puppy and Kitten Problems

*By Dr. Randy C. Lynn, Summerfield, North Carolina*

Considering the complexity and size of the skin (it is one fourth the total body weight of a newborn puppy) and the amount of genetic tinkering that dogs and cats have survived over thousands of years, it is not altogether surprising that something goes wrong once in a while. In general, we know that dogs have been more thoroughly bred for certain characteristics than cats have, resulting in greater variety among dog breeds than cat breeds.

The basics of genetics state that if you select and breed for a certain desired feature, then you unknowingly breed for other *undesirable* features. With dogs that have been bred with an eye on one or two physical traits, there is a higher chance for an undesirable skin disorder to creep in unexpectedly. That's why mixed breed dogs are less likely to suffer from genetic or hereditary diseases than many of the purebreds. As for cats, which have been subjected to less selective breeding pressure, there is less likelihood of genetically related skin problems popping up. In some cases, a genetic or hereditary "disease" is in fact the trait that makes a particular breed valuable. Take, for instance, the Chinese crested and Mexican hairless dogs. They are examples of a genetic disease giving the breed its unique look.

The goal of this chapter is to document the biology of these disorders as they relate to the dogs and cats, not to pass judgment on particular breeds. For the purposes of this discussion, "pediatric diseases" consist of the skin diseases of young puppies and kittens. They include disorders caused by the external environment (nutrition, bacteria, parasites, etc.) and the internal environment (genetics, hormones, etc). "Congenital diseases" include conditions where the young animal is malformed at birth, due to non-genetic problems when the fetus is growing and developing. For example, we know that if a pregnant animal is given certain drugs, the pups will be malformed, even though they will have normal genes. If they are bred, these malformed dogs will have normal offspring. Finally, "hereditary disorders" include those conditions where the genetic makeup of the animal is abnormal. This trait is passed on to subsequent generations.

# Pediatric Skin Conditions

Not enough is known about the real root of pediatric skin disease — whether it is caused by infectious, congenital or genetic abnormalities. The experts agree, however, that many of these conditions are suspected to be genetic. In those cases of genetic disease, it is suggested that affected animals and their parents should be eliminated from all future breeding programs. When in doubt, don't breed these animals. Fortunately, the most common congenital skin disease of dogs and cats is not considered genetic.

### Juvenile Cellulitis

This disease is most common in short-haired dogs between three and 12 weeks of age. Juvenile cellulitis — which is also known as puppy pyoderma, juvenile pyoderma, and puppy strangles — is often considered the canine equivalent of "zits" in teenage children. The syndrome is probably due to a mixture of causative factors including hormone changes, nutritional imbalances, stresses due to parasites, and poor hygiene. These factors must all be addressed when formulating a plan for treatment. The condition consists of small pustules, mostly around the face and head, but also occasionally on the ears, abdomen, prepuce, and around the rectum.

These pustules rupture easily and ooze serum and pus, which dries to form a tan crust. The lesions are usually deep and cause permanent scarring. Bacterial cultures of the pus usually fail to grow any bacteria, or may grow only normal staph bacteria. In the early stages of the disease, puppies are otherwise normal with a normal body temperature. In the later stages of the disease, in severely affected dogs, septicemia may develop with fever, anorexia and depression. In most cases the lymph nodes nearest the pustules are swollen and inflamed. When the lymph nodes in the throat become enlarged it looks as if they will strangle the puppy, thus the origin of the term "puppy strangles."

Topical treatment of this condition must be done very gently, and the urge to "pop" the pustules must be resisted. Vigorous scrubbing and irritation of the lesions can result in extensive and permanent scarring. The best topical therapy consists of warm water soaks in Burow's solution for 5-10 minutes, three to four times daily. While topical therapy is helpful, real relief is only possible with high-dose systemic corticosteroid and antibiotic therapy. Improvement usually is noticeable within 48 hours of therapy, and complete recovery usually occurs soon after.

Caution: It is critical that the veterinary diagnosis is correct, because if the real problem is a severe bacterial or parasitic condition, corticosteroids can bring a problem from bad to worse. Even after a rapid recovery, the medication should be continued for at least two weeks longer to affect a cure. The condition does not usually recur after maturity.

### Infantile Pustular Dermatosis

This is a somewhat similar pustular disorder which occurs in very young puppies up to three weeks of age. It occurs less commonly than juvenile cellulitis. Puppies affected by infantile pustular dermatosis have small pustules which progress to small yellow, reddish or brown crusts. These puppies have a normal temperature but will not eat. Puppies with the most severe form of the disease will die if not treated quickly. Treatment with a combination of antibiotics and corticosteroids is most often successful. In these young puppies the length of corticosteroid therapy should be kept to minimum. We now must consider some of the less common but more interesting disorders which are considered primarily genetic in origin. Several of these diseases have only been described in a handful of animals.

### Cutaneous Asthenia

This skin problem also goes by a number of other names: Ehlers-Danlos Syndrome, Rubber Puppy Disease, Dermal Fragility Syndrome, Dermal Collagen Dysplasia and Dermatosparaxis. Cutaneous asthenia appears to be a genetic disorder which has been described in dogs, cats, sheep, cattle, mink and ... people. Cutaneous asthenia is characterized by skin that is very loose to the body, hyperextensible (like rubber), and very fragile. These animals are most usually covered with open wounds, produced by activities that would produce no lesions in the normal animal. For example, scratching at an ear normally produces no observable reaction, but in a dog with cutaneous asthenia the result is an open wound where the fragile skin has been torn.

Close examination of the skin reveals that it is as thin as cigarette paper, and rubbery enough to allow it to be stretched away from the body much more than normal. The underlying problem is that the collagen bundles fail to form normally.

In normal skin, the collagen bundles act like rubber bands to give the skin its strength and elasticity. Without normal collagen, the skin is easily torn. The disease is incurable. Affected animals should be protected from all possible injury. Special protection is needed to prevent injury during normal daily activity. Declawing the hind feet of cats can help prevent laceration by the hind claws. All cuts must be promptly sutured and protected until they are completely healed.

### Primary Acanthosis Nigricans

This genetic disorder affects only one breed: the dachshund. A similar disease in people is known to be inherited. Acanthosis nigricans produces lesions unlike any other disease. Once you've seen it, you never forget it. Affected dogs begin showing hyperpigmentation (blackening) of the skin in the armpits, followed by a thickening of the skin, and hair loss. It looks almost like the dog has big chunks of tar stuck under the armpits. Eventually the condition spreads to the groin, elbows, hocks, under the tail, around the eyes, and the ears.

Biopsies of the skin reveal that the epidermal layer is hyperplastic (thickened), and more importantly there is an overproduction of melanin pigment. Veterinarians do not normally rely upon the skin biopsy for a final diagnosis, because the skin can have the same visible reactions to several other irritants. But the biopsy must nevertheless be performed, and the results studied along with the physical examination, breed and age of onset. Only when all these factors have been considered can the veterinarian make a diagnosis of acanthosis nigricans.

Primary acanthosis nigricans is the result of a genetic defect which produces the horrible tar-like lesions. This is what separates primary acanthosis nigricans from secondary acanthosis nigricans.

### Secondary Acanthosis Nigricans

This affliction is not genetic in nature, but results from the skin's reaction to a variety of "insults." It is not genetic in nature, although the final results look pretty much the same: thickened, blackened skin. Common causes of secondary acanthosis nigricans include skin friction in obese dogs, hormone abnormalities, and allergies to pollens, foods or contact allergens. Because primary acanthosis nigricans is genetic in origin, there is no cure, but it can be controlled with melatonin injections. Evidently, melatonin (a hormone produced by the pineal gland in the brain) has some positive effects on the overproduction of melanin, a black skin pigment. Systemic corticosteroids and vitamin E therapy have also been reported to help control the clinical evidence of the disease.

### Familial Canine Dermatomyositis

This is an inflammation of the skin and muscles of young Shetland sheepdogs and collies, known to be caused by a genetic abnormality. (See page 165 for a complete discussion of this disorder.)

### Acral Mutilation Syndrome

An unusual disease, Acral Mutilation Syndrome has been reported in German shorthaired pointers and English pointers. It is definitely genetic in nature. The disease is characterized as a defect in the sensory nerves of the feet. It usually becomes apparent in pups from three to five months old, which furiously lick and chew at their feet. The hind feet are often worse than the front feet, swollen and damaged from the abuse. A close examination will reveal that the feet are totally numb.

If the dogs are allowed to continue gnawing at their feet, they will eventually completely amputate their toes and parts of their feet. But because of the numbness, they will still walk without discomfort on the mangled feet or the remaining stubs. Attempts to bandage and protect the feet from trauma are uniformly unsuccessful, and euthanasia is usually requested when the feet are mangled beyond hope of salvage.

### Acrodermatitis

This is an uncommon genetic disorder reported in bull terriers. In fact, it is a genetic defect in the ability to absorb and metabolize zinc. This condition affects many organ systems throughout the body, in addition to the skin. Puppies are born with lighter than normal skin pigmentation, and they grow slower than their litter mates. Soon after weaning they are sluggish and spend much of their time sleeping.

The average dog survives to seven months of age; nearly all die by 15 months. The skin lesions typically are crusts and ulcers on the ears and muzzle; papules and pustules may be found around the body orifices and especially on the head. The feet are also affected by pus between the toes and around the claws. Later on, there are changes in the footpads with excessive growth of rough pad areas and malformation of the claws. All affected dogs die because of serious defects in the brain and severe bronchopneumonia. Every attempt should be made to prevent continuation of this genetic trait.

### Dermoid Sinus

The dermoid sinus has been reported in the Rhodesian ridgeback dog, shih-tzu and the boxer. It is a genetic defect in the development of the puppy, resulting from the improper development of the fetal neural tube, which is supposed to develop into the spinal cord and spinal column. However, the tube splits during development and the dog is born with a small tube in the upper neck which runs from the spinal cord to the skin. This tube varies in length. In some individuals it may run from the skin completely into the spinal cord, while in others it may be just a short hair-filled sinus in the skin. Dogs with this defect should have a complete physical examination, including X-rays of the sinus to see how deep it goes. If it is deep, it should be surgically removed to prevent serious problems in the future. Affected dogs should not be used for breeding.

### Chediak-Higashi Syndrome

This genetic disease has been reported in smoke-colored Persian cats, white tigers, Hereford cattle, Aleutian mink ... and people. It is caused by a defect in the formation of the black pigment granules of melanin. All affected animals have light coat colors and light-colored eyes. The disorder predisposes cats to infection by bacteria, viruses and fungus. There is no treatment.

### Color Mutant Alopecia

This genetic problem has also been termed blue Doberman syndrome, fawn Irish setter syndrome, and blue dog disease. It has been reported in blue, red and fawn Doberman pinschers, fawn Irish setters, blue dachshunds, blue chow chows, blue standard poodles, blue great Danes, blue Italian greyhounds, and blue whippets. In fact, virtually all dogs with this color pattern are affected by the problem. The dogs are born with normal skin and haircoat, then as they get older they develop a thin haircoat, and the skin becomes dry and scaly. Only the blue portions of the coat are affected, and the normally pigmented areas seem to be normal. Later, papules develop in the affected areas, and may develop into pustules. The sole treatment is topical shampoo therapy to help control the papules and make the dog comfortable. The hair does not regrow, and all reported therapy has been unsuccessful.

### Feline Alopecia Universalis

This occurs when cats have the genetic inability to grow primary hairs. This is the breed standard for the Sphinx cat, although it has also been reported (albeit rarely) in other breeds. These cats may have small numbers of downy secondary hairs, but the long straight thick primary hairs are totally absent. Cats with feline alopecia universalis cannot groom normally and must be bathed twice a week by their owners. They are otherwise normal, and are highly prized as breeding animals.

### Canine Alopecic Breeds

There are several well-recognized dog breeds from all over the globe that are characterized by various degrees of alopecia or baldness. These dogs have been selected for centuries to fix this genetic trait into the breed. While biologically abnormal, they are normal for that breed. More specifically, we are referring to the Chinese crested dog, the Mexican hairless, the chihuahua to some degree, the

Abyssinian dog, the African sand dog, the Turkish naked dog, the Peruvian hairless dog and the Xoloitzcuintl.

### Pattern Baldness

An inherited condition most often seen in dachsunds, pattern baldness often begins at less that one year of age. In males the hair on both ears gets progressively thinner until they are completely bald in the mature dog, while females experience a thinning and eventual baldness on the belly and chest. In females the condition is sometimes confused with estrogen deficiency. Recent research work has shown that some of the new anti-baldness drugs for people may be beneficial in pattern baldness dogs.

## Look Long Before You Leap

There are many other genetic disorders that have been described in a few animals or in uncommon breeds, but space precludes their coverage in this text. Advanced veterinary textbooks and scientific articles should be consulted for more information about those disorders. In most cases, the diseases discussed in this chapter should be avoided whenever possible by careful selection and breeding. In others the genetic abnormalities have been selected and fixed into the genes of the breed, becoming the most valuable asset of the breed.

# Canine Dermatomyositis

*by Dr. Ann M. Hargis, Edmonds, Washington*

Canine dermatomyositis is an inflammatory condition of the skin, muscle and sometimes blood vessels. The problem typically afflicts collies and Shetland sheep dogs (shelties), and rarely has it been seen in other canine breeds. Dermatomyositis is widespread and well-documented in collies, but less is known about the condition in Shelties. The disease usually develops in young dogs between two and six months of age, although there have been reports of dermatomyositis in adult animals.

Dermatomyositis also develops in humans, juvenile and adult alike. The juvenile form of human dermatomyositis is most like dermatomyositis in dogs. There is inflammation of skin, muscle and sometimes vessels. There are also reports of dermatomyositis developing in identical twins, or in a father and daughter, but usually familial tendencies are less apparent in human dermatomyositis than in dogs.

# Causes

Breeding studies in collies suggest there is an autosomal dominant inherited component in dermatomyositis. This means that dermatomyositis develops in both males and females (autosomal) and that only one parent needs to be genetically affected to pass the disease to offspring (dominant). Not all genetically predisposed dogs develop symptoms of the disease, suggesting that in addition to the inherited component, there are other factors that influence disease development. Environmental factors, for instance, may also play a role in triggering the onset disease or affecting the severity of the ailment. Some of the environmental factors may include viruses, sunlight, hormones and stress. In children, viruses are thought to be one of the more important triggering factors. It is still not known exactly what causes the skin and muscle damage.

The disease is thought to be *immune-mediated*, which means that the dog's immune system actually contributes to the damage. Immune complexes (a bound unit of an antibody and antigen, possibly a virus) have been identified in affected dogs, and are detected before or concurrent with the development of skin disease—thereby suggesting that the immune complexes may be partially to blame for the lesions.

# Clinical Findings

Dermatomyositis can be very mild, moderate or severe. The condition may get better and worse again periodically throughout its course. Dogs with dermatomyositis develop lesions on the face, tips of the ears, tip of the tail, on the feet, and on parts of the legs over the bony prominences. Not all areas are affected in all dogs, and the skin lesions may be more generalized in more severely affected dogs. The lesions consist of areas of hair loss, redness, ulcers, crusts (scabs) and — more rarely — small blisters. In the mildly affected dogs, the lesions may heal, leaving no evidence they were present. When the lesions of moderately or severely affected dogs heal, they may leave behind permanent areas of hair loss (scars), and changes in the skin pigment (lighter or darker color). Some dogs have lesions throughout their lives.

Muscle disease may not be apparent in mildly affected dogs, while more moderately or severely affected dogs lose muscle mass—meaning the muscles become smaller. The loss of muscle mass is most noticeable on the top of the head and in the jaw muscles. In the most severe form of dermatomyositis, which is uncommon, the severely affected dogs may not be able to open or close their mouths more than one or two inches. Also, in more severely affected dogs, the muscle of the esophagus (the tube which leads from throat to stomach) may be affected. The loss of muscle in the esophagus prevents the food from being moved quickly to the stomach. Food may be regurgitated, and some dogs actually inhale pieces of food into their lungs, causing a type of pneumonia (aspiration pneumonia). In more severely affected puppies, growth may be stunted.

## Diagnosis

The diagnosis of dermatomyositis is made by a variety of factors in combination, and by ruling out the presence of other diseases that may affect young dogs and that can look similar. Unfortunately, there is no one specific test that can be performed to make the diagnosis of dermatomyositis. The location on the lesions (lesion distribution) is fairly unique, which is helpful. Also, skin and muscle biopsy samples (small pieces of skin and muscle) collected for evaluation by a pathologist are also very useful. In addition, there is a muscle test called the electromyogram (EMG) which is similar to the test used to evaluate heart function, the EKG. Dogs with dermatomyositis have some EMG changes that can be very suggestive. Taken together, these tests often lead to the diagnosis of dermatomyositis.

## Differential Diagnoses

The diseases that need to be ruled out include demodicosis (a mite infestation which can be present concurrently with dermatomyositis), dermatophytosis (ringworm), bacterial skin infections, juvenile pyoderma (a non-infectious disease that looks like a bacterial infection), and immune-mediated diseases such as lupus erythematosus and polymyositis.

## Therapy

Because dermatomyositis can get better and worse on its own, and because some dogs are mildly affected while others are more severely affected, it has been difficult to judge the effectiveness of different therapies used for dermatomyositis. Hypoallergenic shampoos are generally beneficial. It is also helpful to keep affected puppies on a soft, clean and dry surface so their skin is not traumatized. Neutering the animals is important not only because the disease has an inherited component, but because in female dogs the hormones may cause the disease to worsen. Sunlight also makes the disease worse, so it is important to keep the affected dogs out of direct sunlight, especially during the summer months and midday hours.

The oral medications thought to be helpful include vitamin E (100 to 400 IU/day) and glucocorticoids (steroids). Most dogs affected seriously enough to require therapy are started on a higher dose of glucocorticoids (1 to 2 mg/kg orally every 12 hours), and when the dog begins to respond to treatment, the dosage is reduced gradually and given on an alternate day basis to reduce any side-effects. There is also an experimental drug, pentoxifylline (Trental—Hoechst-Roussel) used by some dermatologists, but the optimum dose necessary to control canine dermatomyositis has not been established.

## Prognosis

The outcome for an individual dog is difficult to predict because some dogs are mildly affected, while others are more severely affected. Prognosis for long-term survival in mild and moderately affected dogs is generally good. Minimally affected dogs recover spontaneously (with no medications) and heal without scarring. Mildly to moderately affected dogs may also recover spontaneously, but usually have permanent areas of hair loss and color changes in the skin, most notably on the face. Secondary infections with bacteria and demodectic mites need to be treated. Prognosis for long-term survival for severely affected dogs is poor. These dogs tend to have continued skin and muscle disease, including the involvement of the muscles used to chew, drink and swallow. Aspiration pneumonia is a risk in these dogs.

# Sebaceous Adenitis (SA)

*By Dr. Steven A. Melman, Potomac, Maryland*

A disease which affects certain prevalent breeds, sebaceous adenitis is often noticed by the alert groomer first. Since most of what we know about SA comes from case histories of standard poodles, this discussion will focus on the disease as it occurs in this breed. Other breeds, notably the Akita, Samoyed and vizla, presumably have an identical disease. Sebaceous glands seem to be attacked selectively by inflammation to the point of destruction. In advanced cases, the hair and surrounding appendages are also involved. Diagnosis is often clearly confirmed through properly selected skin biopsies. However, some early or mild *subclinical* cases may not show signs of disease on a particular biopsy, and the choice of an area, lesion or biopsy site is critical. So it is difficult to consider a standard poodle "normal" simply by examining a single biopsy. Recent research indicates that SA is most likely an autosomal recessive genodermatosis. This means that if two *subclinically* affected animals are bred together, then each offspring will develop SA. It is important to note that while some dogs have severe clinical signs, the signs in others are so mild that they can only be identified by biopsy.

## Clinical Signs

Young- to middle-aged dogs are usually affected, and there is no gender preference. Long and short-coated breeds may be affected.

The standard poodle, Samoyed and Akita have the long-coated form. As previously described, standard poodle is the best breed to study, possibly because it is most likely to visit the pet professional—pet stylist/groomer. First reported in the black and apricot colors, SA now is seen throughout the breed. The first signs are excess scaling, and dry, brittle hairs, with partial hair loss usually first noticed along the dorsum. Frequently affected areas include the back of the neck, top of the head, nose, trunk and pinnae (ear flaps). Usually, there is no itch or smell. Often, SA does not progress any further.

Cases that progress develop follicular casts or tightly adherent silver-white scales along the hair. These cases may lead to secondary infection, becoming itchy and developing an odor. Oddly, some cases heal spontaneously and then recur, in a cruel cycle independent of treatment. Akitas seem to have a more severe variant of the disease. Dogs which do not have clinical signs but do show signs of disease on biopsy are called "subclinically affected." In short-coated breeds such as Vizlas, the initial signs include circular areas of hair loss that look moth-eaten, with mild scaling primarily affecting the trunk, head and ears. It usually doesn't itch, and no secondary skin infection occurs. The most common differential diagnoses are seborrheic skin diseases and pyodermas (skin infections). Other differentials include demodicosis, ringworm, endocrine disorders and cheyletiellosis. The pet's history will reveal a failure to respond to conventional therapy, both topical and systemic.

## Diagnosis

History, clinical signs and a breed's prevalence lead to a diagnosis which can be definitively confirmed via histopathologic examination of a properly taken skin biopsy. All biopsies from standard poodles—with specific AKC registration number—should be forwarded to *Genetic Disease Control (GDC) in Animals, PO Box 222, Davis, CA 95617, 916-756-6773.* An open registry has been created which allows availability of this information to any breeder who requests it. Due to the difficulty of declaring an animal normal, this is the only type of registry that could be established. If a dog 18 months or older has a history of SA, or if its owner plans to breed it, then the animal should be registered. To do so, have two 6mm punch biopsies sent to a GDC-participating pathologist. It is important to register ALL dogs with the disease, even if they are not intended for breeding. The minimal charge for registration is waived in affected dogs. Dogs less than five years old should be biopsied every year; those five and over, every other year. The biopsy area should be the dorsal cervical area in normal dogs, and the affected areas in affected dogs.

Biopsies can be interpreted as "affected," "questionable," or "normal." "Affected" is self explanatory, but "normal" can be confusing. It does not mean the dog is not a carrier or will never get SA. It just means the biopsy shows no signs. "Questionable" is designated for cases where lesions are present but too subtle to allow a definitive diagnosis. This can occur in the early stages, in the mild form or in any skin disease that can be confused with SA. These cases are sent to a second pathologist for confirmation. All standard French poodles should have their registration checked before breeding.

## Treatment

Remarkable results have been obtained recently in treating short-coated breeds with the retinoid etretinate (Tegison), if treatment is initiated early enough. Other cases remain largely unresponsive. Some have used anti-seborrheics, emollients/humectants and dietary fatty acid supplements. All are useful in mild cases but offer little benefit in advanced cases. Two other treatments have been mentioned to treat these advanced cases. They are: (1) topical application of a high concentration of bath oil and water applied once daily as a spray; and (2) high dosages of essential fatty acids. I prefer to use a full-body application of DermaPet Conditioner, or Oatmeal Conditioner if itching is present, allowing the product to dry on the affected areas. Others have used Alpha Keri Oil as well to add moisture in the horny layer of the skin.

Old literature mentions the use of propylene glycol, but this may have adverse side-effects. Some high-dose topical oil applications require the use of a shampoo to remove the oily residue. High-dose fatty acids—evening prim-rose oil or others produced by various companies—can occasionally be beneficial, although side-effects, including vomiting, flatulence and diarrhea, can occur.

Response to corticosteroids has been unrewarding. However, the use of synthetic retinoids, mainly etretinate (Tegison) but also isotretinoin (Accutane), has been helpful. Cyclosporine (Sanimmune) has been effective in some refractory cases. Basic symptomatic treatment of associated secondary problems, such as skin infections and supportive topical therapy (see Shampoo Therapy, Chapter 4) is important, as with any skin condition. In general, response to therapy is quite variable. The short-coated cases do best, while the akita is the most difficult.

*Robert Dunstan DVM, MS provided special assistance for this article. Further information can be obtained from Progress in SA Research, available from the Genodermatosis Research Foundation, 1635 Grange Rd., Dayton, OH 45432.*

# 11

# KERATINIZATION DISORDERS / SEBORRHEA

*By Dr. Dunbar Gram, Virginia Beach, Virginia*

A ll skin undergoes the process of keratinization, as do several other structures such as the hair and nails. The term keratinization refers to the normal process in which a living immature epidermal cell moves from the deepest part of the epidermis toward the surface, and undergoes a biochemical process in which keratin is formed and the cell dies. Keratin is a unique protein that adds structural support to the skin, and functions to decrease the passage of substances such as water and other compounds into and out of the living organism. The time in which the normal cell takes to go from the lower level of the epidermis to its final death, is called the *epidermal turnover time*. In a normal dog, the epidermal turnover time takes about 22 days.

Under normal conditions, this process would not be noticeable. It's nature's way of getting rid of the old, and bringing in the new. But when the process of keratinization is hit with a defect, the result can be seen in a variety of scale formations — ranging from a fine scale visible as "dandruff," to a thick crust that looks like small sticky flakes. Hair and nails may or may not be involved in this ailment.

Keratinization defects can be divided into two broad categories:

•**Secondary keratinization disorder**. This is when an underlying disease is causing the abnormality. Typical underlying causes include allergies, ectoparasites, ringworm, bacterial infections, hormonal abnormalities (including excess corticosteroid use), cancer, immune mediated (auto-immune) diseases, nutritional abnormalities and dry ambient humidity.

•**Primary keratinization disorder**. This is when the defect is a primary result of the "system" simply having gone awry for a number of reasons not related to another illness. To veterinarians, primary keratinization defects include idiopathic seborrhea, vitamin A responsive dermatosis, epidermal dysplasia (in West Highland white terriers), schnauzer comedo syndrome, canine ear margin dermatosis and acne.

This chapter will briefly examine these primary disorders, providing the pet owner information on how to recognize and treat (under professional guidance) each ailment.

# Seborrhea

Seborrhea (literally an excess flow of sebum) is primarily a chronic and frustrating nemesis of dogs, and less often of cats. The clinical signs of seborrhea vary greatly among individuals. Some affected animals may look like they have a case of "dandruff" (*seborrhea sicca*), while others will have "greasy" or oily skin and hair (*seborrhea oleosa*). With seborrhea oleosa, a foul odor can be detected. The ears can often be included in this affliction, and occasionally small accumulations of waxy material can be found attached to the hair and skin. Another sign of seborrhea oleosa can be circular crusty "scabs." In a severe case of seborrhea oleosa, the skin can become red and inflamed. Areas of hair loss and itching may also be noted.

The healthy canine epidermal (basal) cell needs approximately three weeks to mature (previously explained as epidermal turnover time) from the deepest part of the skin to the uppermost layer. Seborrhea speeds up this process, cutting the typical three weeks down to one week. What results is an excess of skin cells on the surface of the epidermis, all of them waiting to die and be sloughed away. The presence of so many "corneal cells" results in the appearance of scales, or "dandruff." Occasionally, an oily or greasy hair coat is evidence of a secondary infection, as yeast or bacteria take advantage of the altered skin condition and likewise overpopulate the epidermal outer layer. These bacteria and yeast are present on normal skin, but they get out of control when the keratinization process goes awry. It is these microscopic creatures that cause the bad smells so often associated with seborrhea.

It is very important to note that *most* animals with seborrhea have an underlying disease which contributes to the skin abnormality. When seborrhea is caused by another ailment, it is then known as "secondary seborrhea." The typical underlying factors include allergies (Chapter 8), hormonal imbalances (Chapter 9), parasites (Chapter 7), bacterial infections (Chapter 5), fungal infections (Chapter 6) and tumors (Chapter 18). Once the underlying disease has been diagnosed and brought under control, the skin should return to normal. Consequently, secondary seborrhea has a better prognosis than primary seborrhea.

For those unfortunate animals that have no underlying reason for their seborrhea — those afflicted with primary or idiopathic seborrhea — the road to recovery is much more bumpy. Idiopathic seborrhea is the direct result of malfunctioning epidermal cells, an inherent abnormality for which there is no known cause. Veterinary dermatologists will perform a skin biopsy to confirm that the seborrhea is primary. The veterinarian who performs the biopsy much take care in selecting the appropriate site, and the specimen should be read by a trained veterinary dermatologist or dermatopathologist.

Because therapy for primary seborrhea may be tedious, unrewarding and expensive (not to mention the risk of side-effects), the veterinarian should be absolutely certain that there are no underlying reasons for the seborrhea. Clinical signs usually appear before the pet has reached two years of age. There are also some breeds which are predisposed to primary seborrhea, such as the cocker spaniel, English springer spaniel, basset hound, Chinese shar-pei and the West Highland terrier. These breeds may also suffer from secondary seborrhea, of which allergic dermatitis is a particularly common cause.

If secondary seborrhea is the problem, the underlying disease should be identified and treated. In the meantime, while waiting for the test results to return from the lab, veterinarians will usually turn to a topical treatment (Chapter 4) to control some of the clinical signs. In animals with primary seborrhea, long-term topical and systemic therapy may be necessary. Recently, veterinary dermatologists have used the synthetic retinoid drug etretinate (Tegison$^R$) with some success in treating dogs with primary idiopathic seborrhea.

## Vitamin A Responsive Dermatosis

Some animals that appear to have primary idiopathic seborrhea may actually have a disease called vitamin A responsive dermatosis. This is a very rare disease which has been primarily reported in cocker spaniels. The clinical signs are virtually indistinguishable from those of primary seborrhea, and also often occur before the pet is two or three years old. A skin biopsy read by a trained veterinary dermatopathologist may offer some guidance as to whether or not a patient is suffering from seborrhea or vitamin A responsive dermatosis. While the disease responds to vitamin A supplementation, a dietary deficiency of this vitamin is *not* the cause of the disease. Most likely, there is a localized defect in the skin that affects the skin's ability to use this important vitamin.

A positive response to treatment with a trial course of vitamin A alcohol (retinol) supplementation confirms the diagnosis of this disease. One month or more of therapy may be necessary until any improvement in clinical signs is noted. Full benefit may not be noted until as many as three months of therapy. The supplementation should be continued for the rest of the animal's life.

## Epidermal Dysplasia of West Highland White Terriers*

*Note: This subject is also discussed in Chapter 16.

Perhaps the most severe keratinization disorder seen by veterinary dermatologists, epidermal dysplasia is likely to have a genetic basis, and is only reported in West Highland white terriers. Clinical signs typically appear before one year of age, with erythema and pruritus of the feet, legs and ventrum. Secondary lesions of alopecia, hyperpigmentation (darkening of the skin) and lichenification (thickening of the skin) quickly follow. Quite often, nearly the entire body can be affected. Secondary bacterial and fungal infections are common, with a particular subset of this syndrome being the rapid growth of the *Malassezia pachydermatis* yeast. These organisms can be detected through the epidermal cytology or skin biopsy.

The diagnosis is based on clinical signs and the skin biopsy (which will enable the veterinarian to rule out the numerous other possible causes). Because euthanasia is often considered the only realistic means of relieving an animal from severe and prolonged discomfort, it is of vital importance that the veterinarian thoroughly exhaust all other potential etiologies.

Dogs suffering from the overgrowth of *Malassezia pachydermatis* yeast may respond to treatment with oral and topical ketoconazole. However, the underlying defect in keratinization predisposes the patient to reinfection with the organism. Some animals that are not yet severely affected occasionally respond well to immunosuppressive doses of oral steroids which may be decreased and discontinued in time. The pet owner should realize that this route of therapy may have some serious side-effects, and is not without risks.

## Schnauzer Comedo Disease

As the name implies, the only breed affected by this disease is the miniature schnauzer. Clinical signs usually appear during adolescence. Often, the lesions are discernable by touch before they actually become visible. The top of the back, from the neck to the rump, will have blackheads (comedones) which are sometimes incorrectly referred to as "hives." Crusts and hair loss may also be present, but itching is rare. In some cases, secondary bacterial infections can contribute to the severity of the clinical signs.

Schnauzer comedo disease is thought to be a genetic defect which results in abnormal keratinization of the skin that lines hair follicles. Because it is a genetic defect, there is no true cure. However, the clinical signs can be ameliorated. Veterinarians can also act to deal with the bacterial infections and hormonal abnormalities (especially hyperadrenocorticism) which typically plague dogs with comedones.

Treatment centers around topical therapy with benzoyl peroxide or sulfur- and-benzoyl peroxide shampoos. In severe cases, synthetic retinoids may be used. Many experts may recommend weekly benzoyl peroxide baths to help alleviate the likelihood of recurrent breakouts. Antibiotics may be necessary to treat secondary infections.

## Canine Ear Margin Dermatosis

This is a rare disease that is typically seen in dachshunds and occasionally in other primarily short-haired, long-eared breeds. Early clinical signs include a bilaterally symmetrical appearance of small, tightly adherent greasy plugs affecting the medial and lateral ear margins. The lesions are usually more visible on the portion of the ear farthest from the head. Alopecia of the pinnae may also be present. It is important to note that itching is not a problem with this disease. However, more severe cases will include thick crusts, pain, redness, ulceration and loss of the ear's normal shape.

Canine ear margin dermatosis can likely be classified as an immune-mediated disease. Cushing's Disease may play a role in some patients. Potential underlying causes, or secondary infections, should be identified and treated. If an underlying cause cannot be identified, mild cases can usually be controlled with a combination of anti-seborrheic shampoos and topical steroids. In severe cases, surgical correction may be necessary.

## Tail-Gland Hyperplasia

Similar in appearance to seborrhea, tail-gland hyperplasia will occasionally make its appearance on the area of the tail located some two to three inches behind its junction with the rump. This area of the skin, called the tail gland, is rich in glandular structures and is very prominent in wild dogs. Some speculate this area is a vestigial scent gland. In birds, a similar structure exists: the preen glands. In domestic dogs, the tail gland is rarely visible. Abnormalities of this region can be seen alone or along with seborrhea affecting other areas of the body. Testosterone and testicular neoplasia may also play a role in this disease.

Clinical signs include a palpable and sometimes visible enlargement of this region, which is often accompanied by varying degrees of increased pigmentation, greasiness, scales and hair loss. When secondary bacterial infections occur, large pimples (pustules) may be seen. The disease usually responds to castration, although it may also be alleviated with localized topical treatment and systemic antibiotics (if a secondary infection is present). In cases where castration is not an option, surgery of the affected area may offer an alternative.

## Acne

Teenage humans, adolescent dogs and cats of any age can come down with acne. Some dogs may be naturally predisposed to it, including breeds such as bulldogs, boxers, Doberman pinschers, great Danes, and less often Labrador retrievers and some terrier breeds. These animals may show signs of acne throughout their entire life. Early lesions start as small pimples (pustules) or papules (tiny bumps) that enlarge to the point of rupture. Secondary bacterial infections are common, and sometimes draining tracts and pain are seen. The chin and lower lip are the most commonly affected sites. Other diseases such as demodectic mange and ringworm may have a similar appearance.

Cats can show similar signs at any age, and may also exhibit a "fat chin." Eosinophilic granuloma, ringworm, bacterial infections and demodectic mange (which is rare in cats) may also mimic this disease. In mild cases, treatment is seldom necessary. In more severely affected animals, antibiotics (topical and/or oral), warm compresses, topical benzoyl peroxide washes and occasionally topical steroids are helpful. This area is a good site for topical medication, since it is difficult to lick off. In some cases, benzoyl peroxide may actually cause irritation of an already sensitive area of skin. Several veterinary dermatologists report that refractory cases often respond to the topical use of systemic retinoids such as Retin-A.

# 12

# ENVIRONMENTAL DISEASES

## Burns

*By Dr. Patrick J. McKeever, St. Paul, Minnesota*

**B**urns may be minor and cause little discomfort to a dog or cat, or they may be extensive and result in severe discomfort. Treatment of minor burns is routine and generally offers a good outcome, but treatment of severe or extensive burns is complicated, difficult and not always successful.

### Four Typical Causes of Burns

●*Thermal burns* are the most common type of burn experienced by pets. These occur when excessive heat is applied to the skin. Pets may suffer both minor and extensive thermal burns as a result of home or auto fires, scalding, inappropriate use of heating pads and use of malfunctioning commercial hair drying equipment. A common example is a *clipper* burn, a minor burn that may occur when an overheated clipper blade comes into contact with the pet's skin during grooming. In some cases, a clipper burn is not a true burn but an abrasion caused by the sharp teeth of the clipper blade inadvertently scraping the skin.

●*Caustic (chemical) burns* occur when a substance such as a strong acid or alkali comes into contact with the skin and kills skin cells.

•*Frictional burns* usually occur when an animal is hurled or dragged over the pavement after being struck by an automobile.

•*Electrical burns* usually occur when an animal has chewed on an electrical cord. They are generally noted about the mouths of young animals.

## How Burns Are Classified

In humans, burns are classified as

1) first degree, with redness and damage to skin cells but no blisters;

2) second degree, with formation of blisters and the complete death of superficial skin and some damage to the deeper layers of skin; and

3) third degree, with the death of skin cells in all layers.

These classifications cannot be applied to dogs and cats because their thin skin does not blister as easily as humans' skin. Therefore, it is more practical to use a simplified system that classifies burns according to two types: *partial-* and *full-thickness.*

•*Partial-thickness* burns are characterized by damage to, but not complete destruction of, the most superficial skin cells. Healing is prompted by undamaged cells within the superficial layers of the skin.

•*Full-thickness* burns are characterized by complete destruction of all skin cells, including the nerves. Healing of full-thickness burns occurs when undamaged skin cells migrate from the edge of the wound, or through skin grafts.

It may not be possible to determine the extent or severity of a burn wound until after the dead skin has separated and healing has started. However, it is important to determine the extent and severity of a burn as early as possible, so dead skin cells can be excised or removed. In partial-thickness burns, the skin is red, swollen, sensitive to touch, and there is evidence of blood flow to the skin. In full-thickness burns, there is a lack of blood flow to the skin, the skin is insensitive to touch, and the hair is easily removed.

By estimating the extent of a burn, we can predict what the outcome of the injury will be. A quick way to estimate the extent of a burn is with the *Rule of Nines*: Each forelimb represents nine percent of total body surface area; each rear limb represents two nines, or 18 percent; the head and neck represent nine percent; and the chest and upper back represent 18 percent. Veterinarians agree that a full-thickness burn which covers more than 50 percent of a dog's or cat's body indicates a grave prognosis. In such cases, they usually recommend humane euthanasia.

# Physical Changes Associated with Burns

### Shock

Burn shock occurs when the body's automatic regulating mechanisms are unable to ensure normal blood flow in vital tissues and organs, including the heart, brain, lungs, liver and kidneys. Blood pressure and blood volume begin to fall within minutes after an animal has been severely burned; the lowest values occur within two to six hours. The small blood vessels in burned tissue become permeable due to direct thermal injury, and blood vessels distant from the burn wound become permeable due to the release of vasoactive substances (prostaglandins, leukotrines, histamine, serotonin, kinins, and oxygen radicals) from damaged cells.

Hypovolemic shock, or decrease in volume of circulating blood, can be a serious risk if more than 15 percent of the dog's or cat's body surface area is affected by a full-thickness burn. However, the risks probably are less severe than for humans, because these animals are less prone to develop vesicles and blisters. In addition, the ability of the heart to beat strongly also is impaired due to the release of a myocardial depressant from the burned tissue.

### Blood Disorders

The heat that causes a thermal burn kills a number of red blood cells immediately after the injury. The cell count continues to decrease as the bone marrow, which produces red blood cells, is suppressed. This suppression is thought to occur due to toxic products produced by bacteria that infect the burn wound.

### Respiratory Disorders

Animals that suffer severe burns often have difficulty breathing due to the inspiration, or intake, or hot air and gases that may burn the upper respiratory tract. High temperatures may cause immediate injury to the mucous membranes of the upper airway. In addition, the inhalation of wastes or liquid soluble gases—carbon monoxide, sulfur dioxide, chlorine, nitrous oxide, hydrogen chloride, hydrogen cyanide and aldehydes—can cause caustic or chemical injury, killing cells that line the respiratory tract. Soluble gases also impair the function of red blood cells by preventing oxygen from binding to hemoglobin.

### Liver Disorders

Hypovolemic shock diminishes blood flow in the central portion of the liver lobule, thus reducing the supply of oxygen and causing liver cells to die. If enough liver cells are damaged, liver metabolism will be impaired. As a result, liver glycogen stores will be depleted and blood levels of ammonia, amino acids, phosphates, sulfates and lipids will be elevated.

### Kidney Disorders

Kidney function declines partly due to decreased blood pressure and partly due to the buildup of toxins within the kidneys. The kidneys stop producing urine when systolic blood pressure drops below 60 mm Hg. Therefore, a decrease in urine production may be an early sign of kidney damage in severely burned patients.

### Metabolic Alterations

Until burn wounds are healed or grafted, burn patients have increased metabolic rates (one-and-a-half to two times above normal) and often lose weight. The metabolic rate increases as the body tries to compensate for protein loss and heat loss.

### Bacterial Infection

Infections are caused by opportunistic microorganisms found among the normal microflora or environment of the skin. The damaged tissue of the burn wound acts as a medium to support bacterial growth at the same time that the host's defense mechanisms against infections are impaired. In the week following a burn injury, the wounds are colonized by bacteria normally found on the skin as well as exogenous gram-positive flora. During the second week, exogenous and endogenous gram-negative bacteria become prominent. Posing the greatest threat are (1) group A B-hemolytic *Streptococci*; (2) penicillin-resistant hemolytic *Staphylococcus*; and (3) *Pseudomonas aeruginosa*. *Pseudomonas spp*, the most frequently cultured bacteria of burned skin, have the potential to cause a serious infection because they often are resistant to almost all antibacterial agents. In fact, they may cause death in an animal even though there is no increase in white blood cell count, fever, or positive blood culture as is typical in other organisms.

Systemic complications can arise from bacterial infections, although they are rare in small- and medium-sized burns. In extensive burns, where 15 to 30 percent of the body is involved, septicemia (bacteria in the bloodstream) and invasive spread of local infection are common complications. These conditions occur when bacteria proliferate in the necrotic tissues of the burn wound and when these microorganisms penetrate into the bloodstream. Extensive local infection may convert a partial-thickness necrosis into a full-thickness defect. Qualitative bacteriological analysis of burned tissue in humans has shown neither systemic nor topical antibacterial treatments can sterilize a burn wound. However, quantitative methods show that topical antibacterial treatment—but not systemic antibacterial treatment—can significantly reduce the number of microorganisms in the burn wound. Drugs systemically administered apparently have limited or no effect on necrotic tissues.

# Treatment

### Minor Burns

Neither experiments involving animals nor clinical studies involving humans have shown any particular treatment for minor burns to have distinct advantages. If there is minimal redness to the skin but the burn site appears to irritate the animal, a topical anesthetic such as one percent Lidocaine may be used. If there is redness to the skin, a topical steroid also may be used to reduce inflammation.

### Severe Burns

If the burn has occurred within two hours and if the animal permits, ice-water packs (ice and water in a plastic sack) may be applied to the burned areas. Exposed tissue, if present, may be covered gently or wrapped loosely with strips of old sheets or pillowcases. Cooling reduces pain and edema. Skin should be cooled for at least 30 minutes. In dogs, the ideal temperature for the cooling is 3 to 17 degrees Celsius. However, owners should not spend much time with these cooling procedures as they are less critical than a veterinarian's efforts to manage possible shock symptoms.

### Shock

The initial evaluation and treatment of the burn patients is similar to that for animals suffering other severe trauma. Respiratory passages should be examined to assure that the animal may breathe freely. Bleeding should be controlled. Evaluation and, if necessary, treatment for shock should be started (including starting intravenous fluids) according to other articles on this subject.

### Cleaning/Removing Damaged Tissues

To allow for complete inspection of the wound, all hair should be clipped from affected areas. The wound should be flushed with saline or washed with a topical anti-bacterial, such as povidone-iodine soap, to remove hair, dirt and other debris. It can be very difficult to determine the severity and extent of burn wounds in dogs and cats and in general, the area of damaged skin is underestimated. It may not even be possible to delineate the exact area of a full-thickness wound until about 10 days after the injury has occurred, when normal and dead skin starts to separate. All dead skin should be removed as it and any associated fluids provide good growth media for bacteria. Frequent bathing also helps remove loosely attached dead tissue as well as surface exudates. Immersing affected areas in a whirlpool bath for 15 to 20 minutes twice a day is especially effective.

### Topical Treatment

Silver sulfadiazine cream is one of the most effective drugs for killing bacteria in burn wounds. It is non-irritating, easily applied to the burn wound, and reasonable in cost. Except for occasional anemia in cats, it causes no systemic side-effects. After the wound has been cleansed and dead skin removed, the cream is applied liberally to affected areas with a gloved hand or tongue depressor. The wound is then bandaged with loose mesh gauze. This procedure is followed twice daily.

### Skin Grafts

Temporary skin substitutes have been shown to be beneficial as they markedly diminish evaporative water loss, allow host defense cells to ingest and kill bacteria under a protective covering, decrease the pain associated with an open wound, and stimulate the growth of new skin from any remaining epithelial islands. These skin substitutes may be either biologic dressing, such as pig skin, or synthetic skin substitutes made from silicone, polyurethane, or polyvinyl polymers. However, these are minimally effective if there is a lot of bacteria or dead tissue present.

Once all dead tissue has been removed from the wound and infection has been controlled, surgical procedures to decrease the size of the wound may be considered. Dogs' skin is very elastic; its loose subcutaneous tissue allows for considerable stretching. In many instances, skin defects can be closed through direct apposition or one of several reconstructive techniques using skin flaps. If the defect is too large for these techniques to be applied, a free skin graft (either full-thickness or partial-thickness) must be obtained from undamaged skin on another part of the body.

### Systemic Antibacterial Treatment

Studies involving animal and human burn patients have shown that systemic antibiotic therapy does not reduce mortality or fever, or increase the rate

---

## *Frostbite*

### *How Frostbite Occurs*

Frostbite or freezing of the skin is rare in animals. It may occur in cold climates if animals are exposed to sub-zero ( F) temperature for long periods of time.

### *Signs associated with Frostbite*

Skin lesions associated with frostbite or freezing generally are located on the tips of the ears, tip of the tail or scrotum. Frozen skin appears pale, has no sensation and is cool to the touch. After thawing, the skin will become painful and develop varying degrees of redness and scaling. If the freezing was severe, skin cells may die and sloughing may occur. Sloughing often occurs on the tips of a cat's ears; the affected pinnae may curl inward. In addition, hair in areas of skin that has been frostbitten often turns white.

### *Treatment*

If it is unlikely that re-freezing will occur, the affected tissue should be thawed rapidly in warm water (38 to 44 C). If the degree of freezing was minimal but redness and/or scaling are noted, the affected area may be treated with a bland ointment. If lesions are severe and there is sloughing of skin, the affected area should be treated in the same way burn wounds are treated.

---

of healing. Therefore, the use of such drugs probably should be limited to confirmed cases of bacterial septicemia or when quantitative bacterial counts approach $10^5$ organisms/g of tissue. In these cases, the selection of an antibiotic should be determined through culture and sensitivity tests.

# Pressure Sores, Callus, Elbow Hygroma and Photodermatitis

*By Dr. Yasuyo Yamazaki, Chicago, Illinois*

Everybody at some time in their life has experienced some sort of "environmental" skin problem, whether it be a scraped knee or a bad sunburn. The same can be said for our pets, which are just as prone to injuries inflicted by the harsh world we all live in. In this chapter, we'll give a quick look at some of the environmentally related dermatological problems that can afflict domestic pets. You may be surprised at how much we have in common with the tigers and wolves that share our homes.

183

## Pressure Sores

Anybody who has ever cared for a bed-ridden patient knows all about *bed sores*. These "pressure sores" are not to be taken lightly, which is why nurses pay such strict attention to their schedules to make sure immobilized patients are "turned" regularly. Animals, like people, can also fall victim to pressure sores, especially those cats and dogs that are emaciated or so seriously ill that they lay in the same position for countless hours. The first warning sign is a red-to-reddish purple color developing on a small portion of skin covering a bony area. This is the beginning of a common pressure sore, which can all too quickly turn into oozing, dark-colored, or dead tissue. You then have an *ulcer*.

This ulcer can extend well below the visibly discolored perimeter of the wound, much like the base of an iceberg hidden below the surface of the water. What you see of the ulcer may be just the tip of a larger iceberg. The ulcer can also go deep, extending to the bone. What causes this kind of wound? Blame it on excessive pressure, which can cut off oxygen and kill skin tissue, which then becomes infected with bacteria.

The best thing for the animal is to get it back on its feet again, which means taking care of whatever illness or injury put it on its back in the first place. Like any good nurse knows, frequent changes of position (every two hours, if possible) and the use of thicker, softer bedding (such as a waterbed) will help alleviate the development of new pressure sores and promote the healing of old wounds. The wound should be cleaned daily (such as with a whirlpool bath), drying agents, and topical or systemic antibiotics. Healing is slow, and sometimes surgery is necessary to remove dead tissue. In serious cases, skin grafting may be necessary. Throughout the recovery period, your pet must be receiving adequate nutrition. Check with your veterinarian regarding the proper formulations and servings.

## Calluses

Owners of large dogs are usually very familiar with those round hairless areas of gray, rough, thickened, scabbed or wrinkled skin that develop on the animal's hocks or elbows. If you own a dachshund or a Doberman, you may have seen these same thick-skinned areas developing on your pet's chest. If you were worried about ringworm, relax. Your dog is suffering from nothing more than a callus, which results from laying (unprotected) on cement, brick or wood all the time.

You can prevent the growth of calluses, or stop progression in already existing calluses, by providing your pet with a soft place to lay its head. Try foam pads, air mattresses, blankets, etc. A thick-padded protector, such as breeches, may be useful for chronic lesions. If excessive folds or fistulas develop, the solution may include wet soaks or whirlpool baths, topical antibacterial creams (if the callus is infected), and a soothing cream (such as Preparation H) along with frequent bandage changes. Let your veterinarian give you a professional opinion about the severity of your dog's callus problem.

## Hygroma

When the skin covering bony areas is subjected to excessive and unrelenting pressure and injury, it can develop a *hygroma*. This is a red, swollen, fluid-filled, firm-walled cyst that will sometimes ooze when infected. Even if the pet does not seem to be in pain, it most certainly will be once an infection sets in. Fortunately, if you catch the hygroma early enough, you can lessen the injury with softer beddings and by wrapping padded bandages around the wound for two to three weeks. If you do nothing, surgery may become necessary. The hygroma will have to be drained, and in severe cases skin grafting may be needed.

## Photodermatitis

Most of those who once loved sunbathing are now a little more cautious before setting out for the beach, or so we hope. For the past few years, the media have carried numerous warnings about the various bad effects that ultraviolet light can have on our skin, including the development of skin cancers. It doesn't take much for skin to react naturally to sunlight (a tan), and with further exposure or greater ultraviolet light intensities we can easily get hit with a nasty sunburn. But have you ever heard of a *photoallergy*? This is when the skin reacts to a chemical (such as a medication taken internally) that curiously leaves the skin even more sensitive to the damaging effects of the sun's rays. If a substance rubbed on the skin causes a strong sensitivity to sunlight, it is called *photocontact dermatitis*.

In all these things we have a common bond with our pets, for they too suffer from the same potential sun-related problems. That's right, dogs and cats can get a bad sunburn (also called *phototoxicity*) with the same dangers of skin cancer development. Fortunately for our "furry friends," they are far more "furry" than we are. If sun does penetrate the canine and feline fur, their skin reacts in the same way as ours does: They get a tan. A tan is simply the skin's way of protecting itself, as the upper layers of skin darken with melanin to prevent the damaging ultraviolet rays from penetrating too deeply. In a sense, the skin draws the melanin curtains.

But if your animal has a light-colored hair coat, or if your pet has been to the groomer for a very short clip, then you've got to be careful. Dogs with non-pigmented exposed areas, such as the nose, can also get a nasty sunburn. Pay special attention to the risk of sunburn if you live in a sunny climate. Dogs with less pigmentation on the nose can get a condition called *nasal solar dermatitis*. The first signs include a redness at the junction where the hair meets the hairless area of the nose, or the entire nose itself. In severe cases, the nose can become ulcerated and scabbed over. This is rare, but it can progress to a skin cancer.

A dog with short white hair (such as a white bull terrier or a Dalmatian) that loves to sunbathe will get a sunburn mainly on the flank or abdomen, although it can also get burned on the nose, ears or hock. At first, the skin will look red and the dog will seem to experience excessive dandruff. Later, the non-colored skin will become thickened, and upon closer examination you will find cysts, inflammation or blackheads in the hair follicles, along with scarring. Again, this can lead to a later skin cancer.

A cat with white hair (especially one with blue eyes), or a cat with white hair on the ear pinna, is more likely to get a sunburn on its ears. The initial sign is a redness of the skin, starting on the ear margin. As the burn progresses, it becomes thickens, peels, ulcerates and scabs over. It might be itchy and you may see the animal twitching its ears. By the time the margin of the ear curls up, a skin cancer has probably developed which will gradually eat away at the ear. There are many different diseases which mimic phototoxic reactions, so it is important for your veterinarian to make an accurate diagnosis.

An ounce of prevention can save you a pound of cure, so take precautions for your pet's sake. Do not allow animals outside in the sun when the sun is at its hottest, between 10 a.m. and 4 p.m. Animals should be kept indoors, or in the shade. Twice daily, apply a sunscreen with an SPF (sun protection factor) of 15 or more, and if possible get your pet used to wearing a protective T-shirt. You can buy these canine and feline garments from groomers and pet boutique shops. For noses that lack strong pigment, and other de-pigmented areas, use a black felt-tip pen or tattooing to serve as a shading device. If overexposure has already occurred, try applications of topical and systemic steroids, beta-caro-tene (such as Solatene), and synthetic vitamin A (such as Tegison). Other specialized therapy options for those cases which are in danger of progressing to cancer can include hyperthermia, cryosurgery, photochemotherapy, radia-tion therapy, and surgical removal.

So you see, the safest bet is just to keep your sun-worshiping dogs and cats indoors or beneath the shade of some comfortable tree. And while you're at it, make sure you take the same precautions for yourself.

# 13

# NUTRITIONALLY RELATED SKIN PROBLEMS

*By Dr. Lowell Ackerman, Payson, Arizona*

Nutrition is a popular topic among dog owners, breeders and veterinarians, but there are many misconceptions and myths that need to be addressed and corrected. Although nutritional deficiencies can occur, they are actually very rare. More interesting is the fact that nutrients can be used to safely treat a variety of skin disorders in both dogs and cats.

## Essential Fatty Acids

Fatty acids are special chains of carbon atoms to which hydrogen and oxygen atoms are attached. These fatty acids do more than add pounds to our frames. Rather, they are important building blocks for a whole range of important substances, and are needed to maintain normal, healthy cells. Therefore, not all fats are the enemy; some are essential for our health and that of our pets. Fats are common ingredients in dog foods because they make the food much tastier, and because they are "energy dense" — providing over twice as much energy (calories) as either carbohydrates or protein. And yet, dogs and cats have no real fat requirements in their diets. All they need are special fatty acids that are referred to as "essential fatty acids," or EFAs.

These fatty acids are "essential" because they cannot be manufactured by the body, but must be supplied in the diet. The most important members in this class are *cis-linoleic acid, alpha-linolenic* acid and *arachidonic acid.* Cis-linolenic acid is essential for the dog, while cats require arachidonic acid in addition to cis-linolenic acid. Alpha-linolenic acid is not truly essential in people or pets, but is though to be important during certain stages of development.

These EFAs, sometimes referred to as polyunsaturated fatty acids (PUFA), are needed to provide healthy skin and fur, and to promote normal kidney function and reproduction. Fatty acid deficiency is extremely rare in the dog and cat. Most commercial pet foods are high in fats and cholesterol because the typical pet owners want their animals to eat meat — and lots of it! It should be no surprise that where there's meat, there's fat, and the fat is very high in calories. However, commercial rations — especially dry foods — may lose their fatty acid content through the process of "oxidation." That's especially true for foods stored for long periods of time, or exposed to high temperatures.

Rarely, fatty acid deficiency can also result from underlying medical problems, such as liver disease, gall bladder disease, chronic pancreatitis, or chronic digestive disorders. The best way to avoid fatty acid deficiency is to feed a good quality food with adequate fatty acid content. Beware, though, that the body does not need an overwhelming abundance of these fatty acids. In fact, only two percent of the calories needed by dogs should come from EFAs.

In cats, the requirement for cis-linoleic acid is about 2.5 percent of dietary energy, and 0.04 percent for arachidonic acid. The majority of the fat content in pet foods is empty calories from saturated and monounsaturated fats, not EFAs. If necessary, a fatty acid supplement may be purchased commercially, or formulated by adding to the diet small amounts of vegetable oils such as flaxseed, soybean, safflower or corn oil. The best source of EFAs is fortified flaxseed oil, which is low in saturated fats and calories and contains no cholesterol.

In contrast, poor choices are palm, peanut and coconut oils that tend to be high in saturated fats and very low in the required EFAs. Vegetable oil will not meet all the feline's fatty acid requirements, since arachidonic acid is found only in animals. Therefore, a supplement for cats usually contains extracts from meat, fish or egg yolk.

It doesn't take much of these oils to supplement the diet: One teaspoon to one tablespoon daily is sufficient for most dogs and cats. Too much can cause upset stomach and diarrhea, as well as making it difficult for the body to take up and metabolize vitamin E. Caution should be used in giving supplemental fats to pets with medical conditions such as pancreatitis, gall bladder disease, or malabsorption syndromes.

# Active-Form Supplementation

High-quality EFAs may help provide a glossy coat. But also important is that they can be converted in the body into compounds that help relieve inflammation. To accomplish this, however, they must first be converted by enzymes into their *active forms*. Unfortunately, some animals and people lack the enzymes necessary for this process, and so they would undoubtedly benefit from direct supplementation with active-form EFAs.

The active forms of the fatty acids are *gamma-linolenic acid* (GLA), *eicosapentaenoic acid* (EPA), and *docosahexaenoic acid* (DHA). Gamma-linolenic acid is found in several special plant oils such as borage, evening primrose, and blackcurrant seed oil. It belongs to a family called the omega-6 fatty acids. The other two (EPA and DHA) are found in coldwater fish oil, and belong to a family called the omega-3 fatty acids. Most of the benefits from cod liver oil derive from its content of EPA and DHA. These two families of fatty acids perform some very interesting functions in the body.

Oils rich in GLA, when combined with freshwater fish oils, are very helpful for treating inflammatory conditions in dogs and cats. The mixture is commonly prescribed for animals with allergies, but degenerative joint disease (arthritis) and heart ailments might also benefit. It is estimated that 20 percent of dogs with allergies benefit significantly from supplementation with these products. That percentage may not sound like much, but when you realize that these fatty acids have virtually no side effects, it makes sense to supplement.

Most vegetable oils available from pet shops do not contain active omega-3 and omega-6 fatty acids. Look for the proper ingredients on the label: linoleic acid, gamma-linoleic acid; eicosapentaenoic acid; and docosahexaenoic acid. But don't get fooled by imitations. Supplements rich in oleic and palmitoelic acid contain mainly saturated and monounsaturated fats. Supplements containing eicosapentaenoic acid and gamma-linolenic acid are safe and potentially quite beneficial in the management of dogs with allergies and arthritis. It is also possible that eicosapentaenoic acid could be useful for dogs with high blood pressure (hypertension), heartworm disease or other heart ailments. In addition, they provide the EFAs necessary for a shiny coat.

Too much fat supplementation can result in diarrhea and other digestive upsets. Also, do not purchase fatty acid supplements in clear containers, because exposure to light renders essential fatty acids useless. Also be aware that the use of polyunsaturated fatty acids in the diet increases the need for vitamin E. The fish oils that contain the omega-3 fatty acids create more need for vitamin E than the plant-derived omega-6 fatty acids. Any commercial fatty acid supplement purchased should be fortified with vitamin E, and this should be clearly evident in the list of ingredients.

# Zinc

Zinc is a phenomenally important mineral. It is critical in the body's manufacture of proteins and in enhancing the function of enzymes, as well as promoting normal immune functions. Some ingredients in dog foods (e.g., phytates), as well as supplements containing calcium, iron, tin and copper, can decrease zinc absorption. This is one reason why general supplements that include a multitude of nutrients may actually do more harm than good. Anything that interferes with the absorption of zinc, affects its function in the body, or enhances its loss, will reduce the body's stores of zinc.

In recent years, zinc has received much attention. It was documented that some skin diseases in dogs which did not respond to other forms of therapy cleared up entirely with appropriate zinc supplementation. The condition is referred to as zinc-responsive dermatosis, rather than zinc deficiency, because most of these dogs had "normal" levels of zinc in their bloodstream. The more studies that were done, the more it appeared that there may be several reasons for what was observed. Most of the affected animals were sled-dog breeds such as huskies, malamutes and samoyeds. It was felt they might have a genetic defect that results in a decreased ability to absorb zinc from the intestine.

Another group of dogs seemed to have problems that were based in nutrition. For instance, dogs which had been receiving calcium supplements from their owners had problems that would clear up once the supplementation was stopped. In another instance, dogs being fed high-cereal diets were experiencing zinc imbalances. This is because phytates present in cereals interfere with the absorption of zinc. Calcium supplements also interfere with the absorption of zinc from the diet. This seemed to be most acute in rapidly growing breeds, such as Doberman pinschers and great Danes. Yet another closely related problem was seen in dogs fed generic diets. About two to four weeks of eating only generic foods, many of these dogs developed skin problems. They appeared healthy and happy, but they were covered with scabs and sores. Placing them on a diet of quality premium brand name pet foods remedied the problem.

There are many lessons to be learned from these experiences with zinc:

**Proper diet**. It is important for all pets to receive a properly balanced and nutritious diet. This alone prevents many nutritional problems.

**Unwarranted supplements**. The use of high-cereal (high-fiber) diets and supplementation with calcium can impair the body's ability to absorb zinc, even if it is present in adequate amounts in the diet.

**Zinc treatments**. Zinc alone may be a useful supplement when an animal has chronic skin problems or some immune deficiency. And it

190

may be helpful, even when there is no deficiency, because zinc levels are easily lowered by a variety of ailments that might not even be linked to any nutritional problems, such as diarrhea, diabetes, and kidney and liver disease. Zinc also has benefits for the immune system.

There is one other condition that might have something to do with a relative zinc imbalance. Lethal acrodermatitis is a bizarre inherited disease in bull terriers that has many similarities to experimental zinc deficiency. The problem starts in puppyhood, leading to poor growth, skin problems, digestive disorders and recurrent infections. These pups are immunologically crippled, and often die before a year old. The problem is thought to be somehow related to zinc, but supplementation with zinc does not improve the outcome for these poor animals.

Zinc is sometimes used in the treatment of other conditions as well. Recently, it was found that zinc acetate supplementation could be helpful in managing dogs with liver disease caused by copper toxicity. This condition, which is most common in Bedlington terriers and West Highland white terriers has some similarities to Wilson's disease in humans. Although the pattern of inheritance is not precisely known, affected dogs store copper in their livers and eventually poison themselves. Zinc acetate can be used for treatment because it blocks the absorption of copper from the intestines. Previously, only drugs such as penicillamine and trientine were used in treatment, but they have their own unpleasant toxicities. On the other hand, zinc acetate has been used successfully, without any side effects.

However, too much zinc in the diet can cause either diarrhea or constipation, and can affect the levels of other vitamins and minerals. Remember, all nutrients need to be balanced in the body. That's why problems result when we take it upon ourselves to supply one set of nutrients without considering the levels of all nutrients.

## Vitamin A

In many ways, vitamin A behaves more like a hormone than a vitamin. After all, it is not only an important "skin vitamin," but also helps regulate the immune system and promotes a healthier reproductive system and eyes. That's why it is so important that dogs and cats receive vitamin A in their diets. But dogs can also consume beta carotene and convert this into vitamin A. Cats cannot convert beta carotene into vitamin A, and that's why it is so important that their diets include vitamin A rather than the precursor, beta carotene.

As a dietary supplement, vitamin A is especially important for dogs afflicted with a skin condition that is commonly referred to as *vitamin A-responsive dermatosis.* The key word here is "responsive," since this skin condition is not caused by a vitamin A *deficiency.* Rather, this malady responds to *larger doses* of vitamin A than were already present in the animal's diet. This skin condition normally affects the cocker spaniel, but no breed is immune. Signs of the dermatosis include dandruff, hair loss and marked crusting, especially on the back.

The problem should respond to supplementation with megadoses of vitamin A. But be warned: Too much vitamin A in the diet can be harmful. Because it is fat-soluble, vitamin A can accumulate in the liver and cause "vitamin poisoning" if it builds up. That's why it is important that large doses of the vitamin be given only under the supervision of a veterinarian. When treating dogs with megadoses of vitamin A, veterinarians can perform periodic blood tests to guard against any side-effects.

Many supplements designed for skin and immune problems already have considerable amounts of vitamin A, which means you should never add additional vitamin A to these products. When dealing with pregnant animals or those with liver disease, be cautious in the administration of vitamin A. As for felines, vitamin A supplementation is especially risky since their diets already tend to contain large amounts of the vitamin.  ·

# Vitamin E

A natural antioxidant which also acts as a mild anti-inflammatory agent, vitamin E appears to have the most significant effect on the immune system. Supplementation at levels several times above actual requirements can help stimulate an animal's immunity system. Good natural sources of this fat-soluble vitamin include wheat germ, soybeans, vegetable oils, enriched flour, whole wheat, whole-grain cereals and eggs. Adequate levels of zinc are also needed in order to maintain proper levels of vitamin E in the blood.

Naturally occurring vitamin E deficiency has only been reported in cats, usually when their diets contained excessive amounts of canned red tuna or cod liver oil. The result is a potentially fatal condition called *pansteatitis.* Dogs with experimentally induced vitamin E deficiencies showed scaling (dandruff), increased susceptibility to infection, redness of the skin and visual defects (resembling progressive retinal atrophy). This has only been seen experimentally.

In reality, vitamin E deficiency is extremely unlikely for pets that are fed good quality diets. Commercial dog foods, especially dry foods, must add antioxidants to prevent fats from going rancid. Vitamin E can do the job quite well if it is added in sufficient quantities, and if it is not expected to keep food fresh for more than a month or so! Unfortunately, vitamin E is more expensive than chemical antioxidants, and doesn't provide enough preservative power for the many months that a dry food can be expected to sit on store shelves.

In the body, vitamin E is easily affected by other nutrients. For example, excessive supplementation with fatty acids, especially those commercial preparations designed to promote a glossy coat, can actually make it harder for the body to absorb vitamin E. Just another reason why indiscriminate supplementation is not advisable. Vitamin E, which is available in a variety of forms and stabilities, has been used in the treatment of various canine diseases, including discoid and systemic lupus erythematosus, demodicosis, acanthosis nigricans, dermatomyositis, and epidermolysis bullosa simplex. However, vitamin E is rarely successful as the sole element in the management of these conditions. But it is a relatively non-toxic therapy aid.

## The B Vitamins

The B vitamins should seem familiar to almost everybody. This group includes the ever popular thiamine ($B^1$), riboflavin ($B^2$) and niacin ($B^3$). Other important B vitamins include pantothenic acid ($B^5$), pyridoxine ($B^6$) and cyanocobalamin ($B^{12}$). Related compounds are biotin, choline, folic acid and inositol. Deficiencies of B vitamins are extremely rare in dogs, simply because so many different foods contain members of the vitamin B family. There have been reported deficiencies of thiamin in dogs and cats, but these are rare. Most of the problems regarding vitamin B occur in pets that are fed large quantities of raw fish.

Derivatives of niacin have been used to treat skin problems in dogs. In the body, niacin is converted to niacinamide (also called nicotinamide), which then plays a role as part of an enzyme group that helps the body convert nutrients into usable energy. Niacinamide — which is generally available from health food stores and pharmacies — has been used successfully to treat some immune-mediated dog diseases, especially lupus erythematosus. For treatment purposes, it is combined with tetracycline (for its anti-inflammatory effect) on a daily basis.

Other important B vitamins that affect the skin are *pantothenic acid* and *pyridoxine* ($B^6$). Pantothenic acid is known as an "anti-stress" vitamin and helps convert fats, carbohydrates and proteins into energy. It also aids in the formation of antibodies as well as adrenal hormones. Pantothenic acid may help dogs with allergies, as well as those with hormonal disorders. Pyridoxine activates many enzymes, and helps aid the immune system. It also helps maintain sodium and potassium balance, and assists in the formation of new red blood cells. In fact, pyridoxine is probably the busiest of the B vitamins, although it often takes a back seat to thiamin, riboflavin and niacin as far as name recognition is concerned. Pyridoxine is very helpful for animals that need a boost to their immune systems, and for those pets that need a little extra energy while recovering from disease.

Biotin is one of those B vitamins that has received more than its fair share of attention. Even though it is important for healthy skin and fur, biotin deficiencies are extremely rare. Feeding raw eggs to dogs may contribute to biotin deficiencies thanks in large part to avidin, an ingredient in raw eggs that binds biotin in the intestines and prevents it from being absorbed by the body. The danger is removed when the eggs are cooked. There is probably more danger of a biotin deficiency occurring from the chronic administration of sulfa drugs and antibiotics. Biotin is used in the management of a variety of skin diseases, especially those that produce excessive scaling or dandruff.

## Multi-Nutrient Supplements

Pet shop shelves are filled with nutritional supplements for pets, but unfortunately very few of these actually meet the requirements of pets suffering from very specific ailments. As for healthy dogs and cats that are already eating a good balanced diet, supplementation with vitamins and minerals is probably unnecessary. Where these supplements do belong is when pets are living on a steady diet of home-made foods that have not been thoroughly evaluated for nutritional balance and completeness.

Skin diseases are probably the most common conditions for which nutritional supplementation is sought. Although many skin problems benefit from specific supplements, few are the result of actual nutritional deficiencies. A well-formulated supplement will provide high-level amino acids, vitamins and minerals needed for optimal skin care. A supplement that only provides the "recommended daily requirements" will not be enough to achieve those necessary high levels. Most research has looked only at the use of omega-3 and omega-6 fatty acids in the treatment of allergic dogs, but concerned pet owners and veterinarians should also give serious consideration to the use of zinc, vitamin E, the sulfur-containing amino acids and the bioflavinoids.

# 14

# EAR DISEASES AND TREATMENT

*The following is a revised version of articles in Veterinary Forum (July and August 1993) and Groom and Board (September/October 1993) written by the author.*

*by Dr. Steven A Melman, Potomac, Maryland*

The next time you're in a crowded veterinary waiting room, look around at the animals gathered there. Are some dogs and cats shaking their heads, while others are scratching their ears vigorously? Chances are, two out of every 10 dogs in that waiting room is suffering from some sort of ear infection — most likely *otitis externa*, or inflammation of the ear canal. Otitis externa is one of the most common medical problems in canines, accounting for 20 percent of all veterinary visits. Cats are at less of a risk, although anywhere from two percent to 6.6 percent of all feline patients are in for another ear problem — mites (*Otodectes cynotis*). Most of these cases are not life-threatening, but they can be very irritating for the pet, costly for the owner and frustrating for the professional. Sometimes it seems that no matter what treatment is undertaken, the problem just won't go away.

Among these "chronic" cases, as many as 74 percent of the animals may have suffered a ruptured tympanic membrane due to the constant scratching. That leads to more serious problems, because without the tympanic membrane, any fluids and chemicals (even seemingly harmless products such as shampoos) can drip into the pet's inner ear, causing irritation and infection. Veterinarians are

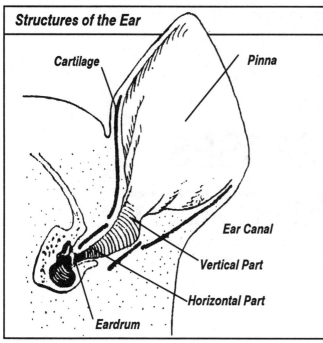

**Structures of the Ear**

Cartilage

Pinna

Ear Canal

Vertical Part

Horizontal Part

Eardrum

*Figure 14.1*

also challenged in these situations, because the fluids they use to clean ears can be potentially ototoxic to the inner ear. For example, the cleaning agents chlorhexidine and salicylic acid are included in many common ear cleansing products, even though these two substances are ototoxic.

Aside from external ear problems, pets may also suffer from difficult-to-treat middle ear problems, such as *otitis media*. Even radical surgery may not be successful in putting things right until the underlying cause has been resolved.

## Causes of Ear Problems

According to John August of Texas A & M University, otitis externa is associated with three types of causes: *predisposing, primary* and *perpetuating*.

### Predisposing factors

Predisposing factors do not actually *cause* otitis externa, but they *increase* the chances that ear problems will develop. The ear, by virtue of its shape, tends to trap moisture, foreign debris and glandular secretions. Excessive moisture causes maceration (softening or thinning) of the skin, which enables the overgrowth of organisms normally found in the ear canal in much smaller numbers. Predisposing factors for ear problems include *excessive hair* (as in the poodle, Old English sheepdog and the Airedale terrier); *pendulous ears* (as in the cocker spaniel); and *narrow vertical ear canals* and/or *folded pinnae* (as in the shar-pei). Contrary to breeders' lore, canine ear hair should be plucked on a regular basis!

### Primary factors

Primary factors actually *cause* otitis externa. Such factors include *allergy* (or hypersensitivity) to foods, substances in the environment, and inhalants; *kera-*

*tinization disorders* such as seborrhea; *parasites* such as ear mites; and *foreign bodies.* (Most of these subjects are discussed in detail in other chapters of this book.)

*Inhalant Allergy:* Common signs of inhalant allergy (atopy) are redness of the pinna and vertical canal, with normal horizontal canals. As a matter of fact, in as many as 20 percent of food allergy cases, otitis externa may be the only sign of trouble!

*Contact allergy:* Although rare, contact allergies may be associated with medications or cleaning agents. You should suspect this whenever an ear gets worse after treatment. Two common culprits are Neomycin and high concentrations of propylene glycol.

*Keratinization disorders:* Endocrine hormonal imbalances (such as hypothyroidism) often lead to the keratinization disorders which can cause a chronic waxy (ceruminous) otitis externa. These conditions are more common among breeds that are prone to seborrhea, such as the cocker and springer spaniels.

*Parasites:* Felines are more likely to suffer from parasite-based ear problems than dogs. In fact, over 50 percent of the otitis externa cases in cats are caused by parasites, while only five to 10 percent of the cases in dogs are a result of parasites. Despite these high numbers for cats, it is still often difficult to find ear mites during a microscopic examination. There are two theories to explain this: There may be only a few mites involved, but the patient is suffering from a hypersensitivity to the invading parasites; or the feline body's inflammatory response to parasitism has driven out the mites. These same explanations have been used to describe scabies (*Sarcoptes scabieii*), another skin disease which often affects the ear as well as other body parts, but with little sign of the parasite causing all the damage.

Other ectoparasites affecting ears less frequently include cat scabies (*Notoedres cati*), *Demodex sp.*, and numerous ticks, including the spiny ear tick (*Otobius megnini*). Microorganisms such as ringworm (*Microsporum canis*) or the *Malassezia* yeast can also be a primary factor in otitis externa.

*Foreign Bodies:* The natural world is full of potential problem-causing foreign bodies, such as plant material (foxtails are common in the West), dirt, loose hairs (especially in short-coated dogs) and dried medication residues.

Other primary causes of otitis externa include glandular disorders, viral diseases, juvenile cellulitis, and autoimmune diseases such as pemphigus foliaceus and lupus erythematosus, which affect the pinna more often than the ear canal.

### Perpetuating factors

Perpetuating factors are those that prevent the resolution of ear problems. These may include bacteria, yeast, progressive pathological changes and middle ear infection (otitis media). Bacteria are not primary causes, but they are secondary problems in that they cause inflammation. One such microbial dilemma is *Pseudomonas,* which is found occasionally in the normal ear or in contaminated water; problems may result from a combination of excessive moisture (such as seen with swimmer's ear) which provides a perfect environment for this common and somewhat persistent ear pathogen. *Staphylococcus, Proteus, E. coli* and *Klebsiella* all may cause secondary problems. Yeast organisms such as *Malassezia* (which is found in 36 percent of normal ears) lead to many of the common complications associated with allergies or antibiotic treatment. In fact, *Malassezia* is most pathogenic when fluid is put into the ears. Progressive pathologic changes include thickening of the skin to the extent that the ear canal becomes closed off or form folds that trap debris and other unwanted organisms. And of course, otitis media can also be an ongoing cause of trouble.

## Clinical Signs

Quite often, the first sign of otitis externa is head shaking (itching). Other common signs include pain, discharge and foul smell, along with head shyness. If the disease progresses, it can lead to head tilting, incoordination (ataxia), Horners syndrome and pain when chewing. Veterinarians often can deduce the cause of otitis externa on the basis of what signs appear first. For example, itching is usually the first sign associated with atopy, foreign bodies or parasitic disorders. Veterinarians also look at the color and odor of the discharge. (See Table 14.1) Finally, veterinarians will consider the animal's medical history and behavioral traits. For example, the professional will want to know if the animal swims often or is affected by changes in the season, or whether the animal has received treatment with irritating products.

When all this information is gathered together with the physical exam, the most common diagnosis usually turns out to be ear mites, foreign bodies or pinnal erythema (allergy). Physical changes — other than the damaged tympanum — may include redness, hair loss (alopecia), scaling, crusting, broken hairs, head shyness and pain. Swelling of the pinna can involve an aural hematoma (the tip of the ear is filled with blood), which must be corrected surgically. Hot spots (also known as acute moist dermatitis) can also occur on or around the pinna.

## Veterinary Care

Once ear disease has been identified and classified, the veterinarian will clean the ear canal and middle ear before applying topical agents and "systemic" therapy (medication). In some cases, a topical anesthetic may be used to relieve moderate pain or irritation. In certain situations, the animal may be sedated during treatment. Selection of an ear cleanser is important. The use of vinegar (either alone or in combination with water or alcohol) has been recommended since the dark ages to treat maladies such as yeast infections. The essential ingredient is acetic acid which, at the proper concentration, can kill *Pseudomonas* in 60 seconds, and *Staphylococcus* and *Streptococcus* in five minutes — not to mention what it does to yeast. The main problem with straight vinegar is that its pH is too low, causing potential problems for canine skin. That's why a product such as DermaPet Ear/Skin Cleanser, which has been pH balanced and

| Organism | Nature of Exudate | | | | | | | |
|---|---|---|---|---|---|---|---|---|
| | Dark brown to black and waxy | Dark brown to black and Dry to powdery | Pale yellow, cheesy | White, creamy to cheesy | Pruritic | Yellow/tan, purulent | Often ulcerative | May smell fruity |
| *Malassezia pachydermatis* (aka *Pityrosporum*, yeast) | + | | | | +/- | | | + |
| *Otodectes cynotis* (ear mites in cats and dogs) | | + | | | + | | | |
| *Psoroptes cuniculi* in rabbits | | + | | | + | | | |
| *Staphylococcus intermedius* or *Strep* Gram negatives, most commonly | | | | | +/- | + | | |
| *Pseudomonas*, less often *Proteus* | | | + | | +/- | | + | |
| *Candida* | | | | + | | | | |

Table 14.1

combined with boric acid for maximum effect and drying, is the choice of many experts for proper ear cleansing — especially in cases of swimmer's ear. Also, this product does not contain alcohol, which can be irritating and dangerous.

Thorough cleaning of the ear is a critical part of treatment — in actuality, it sometimes is all that's needed. Cleaning can remove foreign bodies (which cause the problems in the first place) as well as pus and inflammatory debris (which encourage inflammation and inactivate some medications). Cleaning also makes for an easier exam and enables drugs to reach the affected areas. Veterinarians use a variety of instruments to clean and treat ears, such as a rubber ear bulb syringe, a 12 cc syringe and rubber feeding tubes or urinary catheters cut to various lengths, a suction apparatus, and a water pick. Experts also use curettes, or loops, to remove foreign bodies. Cotton applicators have been criticized as abrasive. Many experts continue to use cotton balls, insisting that these are especially convenient for clients and most effective if not overused. Cotton swabs are too tiny and potentially irritating, and thus should never be used.

## Ototoxicity

Anything that kills nerve cells in the ear — causing deafness and/or loss of equilibrium — is considered *ototoxic*. That doesn't include substances such as

## Ototoxic Drugs

| Ototoxic Drugs | Functional Impairment | Further Information |
|---|---|---|
| Aminoglycosides Gentamycin amikacin, neomycin, tobramycin | vestibular, auditory, both | Concentrate within cochlear cell lysosomes which are found in cochlear hair cells, some hearing loss is delayed until post Tx |
| Erythromycin | both | Labyrinth hyperreflexia |
| Chlorhexidine | inner ear cell | Passes through membranes, both vestibular & auditory in cats |
| Salicylates | auditory | Reversible hearing loss and tinnitus, like nose trauma |

*Table 14.2*

# At-Home Care

***When it comes to cleaning or treating ears, here are a few general guidelines:***
- If the ears are dry, moisten them. If they are wet, dry them.
- Do not use ointments, which generally are occlusive, in moist ears.
- Use easy-to-apply liquids instead of creams to treat difficult areas such as the horizontal canal.

Follow these steps when cleaning ears:
- Apply the recommended amount of ear cleanser into the ear canal and massage thoroughly. Some people temporarily block the canal with a small amount of cotton to prevent the pet from shaking the cleanser out.
- Allow the cleanser to remain in the ear for five minutes.
- Insert cotton wads or balls into the ear and massage the ear so debris sticks to the cotton. An applicator stick may be of assistance where repetitive cleaning is required. In dry and/or irritated ears with little debris and/or wax, a tiny bulb or water pick can be used instead of cotton. When using water, use warm as opposed to cold water for ear cleaning. In severe cases, this process may be repeated from one to three times daily.
- Apply medication, if necessary, after cleaning.

***Pet owners should understand why it is important to clean their pets' ears at home on a regular basis:***

- Many infections can be treated solely through cleaning.
- Serious problems can be prevented from recurring.
- Regular cleaning may eliminate the problem before it has a chance to occur.
- In more serious cases, cleaning can complement systemic and/or topical therapy.

Ear treatments can fail when the veterinarian does not properly explain the necessary treatment and cleaning techniques or does not stress the importance of follow-up care — and when owners do not follow instructions or do not return to have their pets re-examined. Willing and compliant owners, on the other hand, should never have to deal with chronic ear problems among their pets.

water or acetic acid, which can cause a temporary vestibular effect. But aminogylcosides (gentamycin, amikacin, neomycin, tobramycin), erythromycin, chlorhexidine and salicylates (including salicylic acid/aspirin) *are* ototoxic, and in combination their danger is even greater. Therefore, it is especially important to avoid any cleansers and drugs which contain potentially ototoxic ingredients. Clinical signs of ototoxicity include failure to alert, awaken or show reflexes to specific sounds, changes in voice, and unexpected behavior. In humans, tinnitus (ringing in the ears) is often the first sign of ototoxicity, while aging and pre-existing disease seem to also increase the likelihood of adverse reactions to ototoxic substances. It has been noted that the use of calcium and/or antioxidants such as Vitamin E may reduce some ototoxic effects.

# 15

# PODODERMATITIS, EYELIDS AND ANAL SACS

*By Dr. Bill J. McDougal, Houston, Texas*

## Pododermatitis

P ododermatitis, literally inflammation of the skin of the foot, may be caused by infection (bacterial, fungal, parasitic), allergic dermatitis, contact dermatitis, psychogenic dermatitis, autoimmune disease, trauma or idiopathic (unknown) origins. Symptoms include licking and biting at the feet, inflammation, swelling, hair loss, infection and nail-and-pad abnormalities. This syndrome is very difficult to treat effectively because the cause may be multifactorial and obscure.

No breed, sex or age predilection exists; however, it occurs more frequently in breeds such as the basset hound, great Dane, English bulldog, bull terrier, dachshund, mastiff, boxer, weimaraner and shar-pei. Short-coated breeds are affected more often than their long-coated companions. Multiple interdigital areas of one or more feet may be affected. Following are short descriptions of various foot ailments that afflict household pets:

### Bacterial Pododermatitis

Interdigital (between the toes) infection is the most common foot disease, resulting in draining nodules or granulomatous reactions. Cytology and cultures are necessary to identify the cause. Therapy is based on appropriate and usually long-term antibiotic therapy from culture and sensitivity findings. If possible, any underlying causes should be treated.

## Fungal Pododermatitis

Fungal foot infections not only involve the haired portion of the paw, but may also include the nails. Dermatophyte (ringworm) infections are most common, including three strains of the fungus: *Microsporum gypseum*, *Microsporum canis* and *Trichophyton mentagrophytes*. The latter — *T. mentagrophytes* — may be the most common cause of nail infections, followed by *Candida* infections which affect the nail bed area (the paronychia). Diagnosis is based on microscopic examination of potassium hydroxide preparations of hair, scale and nail substance, fungal cultures and histopathology findings. Clinically the diseased nail appears dystrophic (abnormally shaped), broken or split. Generally, involvement of one paw only suggests a fungal, bacterial, neoplastic or traumatic problem. Symmetric (multiple paw) involvement may suggest disorders such as endocrine, autoimmune or nutritional disease.

Treatment of fungal nail disease requires systemic antifungal agents such as griseofulvin or ketoconazole. Some good can come from using topical agents such as iodine or chlorhexidine shampoos and rinses, and antifungal creams or lotions such as chlortrimazole, miconazole or thiabendazole. To clean the animal's housing and sleeping quarters, pet owners can use a chlorinated bleach such as Clorox, although they must be sure the area is completely dry before the animal returns.

## Parasitic Pododermatitis

Demodectic mites are the most common cause of parasitic pododermatitis, leading to secondary infections and swelling of the feet. Diagnosis is based on finding demodicid mites in skin scrapings or biopsies. Treatment requires topical and systemic mitacidal agents such as amitraz or ivermectin. Long-term antibiotic therapy based on culture and sensitivity findings is usually necessary. Hookworm larvae may penetrate the feet and cause pododermatitis. This parasite is more likely to be found with animals living in filth, while those pets exposed to the outdoors may come down with ticks, chiggers and fleas, which also cause pododermatitis.

## Allergic and Contact Pododermatitis

Canines with allergic dermatitis may run the range of pododermatitis symptoms from minor foot licking to the major symptoms of swelling, redness, infection and pain. Allergic dermatitis is caused by a hypersensitivity to inhaled allergens (such as dust, molds and pollens) or food substances. (See Chapter 8.) Less likely, but not impossible, is pododermatitis resulting from contact dermatitis. The area between the toes is the most likely site to be affected by an irritant (such as a chemical) or an allergen (perhaps a plant substance, such as wandering Jew or poison ivy).

## Psychogenic and Autoimmune Pododermatitis

Historically, psychogenic pododermatitis has been more frequent among highly bred and high-strung animals such as the Siamese, Himalayan and Burmese cats, and the German shepherd, golden retriever, Labrador retriever, terrier and poodle. The classical symptom of psychogenic pododermatitis is excessive foot licking, frequently involving only one foot.

Autoimmune disease typically affects the pads of all four feet, resulting in minor symptoms of thickening and scaling, or major signs of severe thickening, fissuring, ulceration, swelling and redness. Other mucocutaneous areas may also be involved. *Pemphigus, pemphigoid* or *lupus erythematosus* can cause pododermatitis. For more details, turn to Chapter 8.

## Traumatic and Idiopathic Pododermatitis

Feet can easily be injured by things such as glass, wire and thorns, which can cause cuts and lead to infection, and potentially, pododermatitis. Secondary problems such as pyogranulomas frequently occur with foreign body (thorns) embedment. The offending agent must be removed. Antibiotic therapy may be necessary in severe cases. In many cases, the cause of pododermatitis may remain a mystery. When faced with this idiopathic pododermatitis, veterinarians may turn to long-term antibiotic therapy, although even this may be to no major advantage. These cases may be frustrating to clinicians and owners. Examples of miscellaneous causes of pododermatitis include zinc-responsive dermatosis, drug eruption or canine distemper.

# Ailments of the Eyelids

Diseases of the eyelid may occur from infection, trauma, anatomical defects, tumors, autoimmune diseases, demodectic mange, allergy (inhalant, food, drug, etc.) and contact dermatitis. More often than not, they are secondary to conjunctivitis and periorbital dermatitis (around the orbit), caused by excessive rubbing. Both dogs and cats have three eyelids: the upper, lower and third eyelid. Only the upper eyelid has a row of eyelashes, while all three have numerous glands, vessels and lymphatics. Not present in humans, the third eyelid is also known as the *nictitating membrane*. It is not covered with an outer layer of skin, projects from the medial aspect (from the nose) of the eye, and protects the eye. Most eyelid diseases also involve the eyeball and other adjacent structures.

This chapter will briefly look at the various diseases of the eyelid.

# Infection

Microscopic organisms such as bacteria, viruses and fungi are the most common causes of infection in the eyelid, eye and periocular areas. But although the irritants may be microscopic, identifying them is a big job. Veterinarians must perform microscopic examinations of skin scrapings, potassium hydroxide preparations, and cytologic evaluation of epidermis and hairs. Cultures for fungal and bacterial organisms may be needed to identify the exact agent causing the infection. Therapy is based upon treating the infection, and correcting any underlying cause.

# Trauma

Primary trauma, or injury to the eyelid, is rare. More likely, a pet injures itself in scratching the itch caused by other illnesses, including eye diseases and larger systemic diseases.

# Anatomical Defects

Some breeds are more unfortunate than others in that they are prone to genetically influenced problems, or defects. The list of susceptible breeds includes shar-peis, St. Bernards, poodles and chows. The typical problems that veterinarians come across most often are:

### Trichiasis

This is an abnormal direction of the eyelashes, as when they eyelashes turn inward and cause a conjunctivitis or corneal abrasion.

### Distichiasis

This is an abnormal position or location of the eyelashes. They may be on the inner eyelid margin, resulting in trauma and infection to the ocular unit.

### Entropion

This is an inversion of either or both eyelids. The lid margins and the eyelashes may cause direct injury to the cornea and adjacent ocular structures. It can only be cured with surgery.

### Ectropion

This is an eversion (turning out) of either or both eyelids. It commonly leads to a secondary infection of the ocular unit, and also requires surgery.

### Cherry Eye

This is an enlargement and infection of the lymphatic gland on the inside surface of the nictitating membrane or third eyelid. The gland may enlarge enough to evert the third eyelid, exposing the inflamed gland that resembles a cherry, thereby giving the illness its name.

### Sty

This is a small inflamed swelling of a sebaceous gland of the eyelid. It may be very painful, and require lancing and topical antibiotic treatment.

### Epiphora

An excess of lacrimation (tearing) can result in a dark red stain on the lower lid, and a secondary infection of the ocular unit. The cause may be a defect in the nasolacrimal system. Surgical correction may be necessary.

## Tumors

Younger dogs do not suffer from eyelid tumors as much as older animals. And while most tumors are benign, they can cause damage to the cornea simply by their location. They can also lead to a secondary infection. Surgical excision may be necessary. But that is not to say that we should assume all tumors are benign. Take no chances, and have the tissue undergo a histopathologic evaluation.

## Autoimmune Diseases

Autoimmune reactions typically occur in mucocutaneous (where mucous membranes and the skin meet) areas, such as the eyelids, lips, ears, genitalia, anus and foot pads. The most common autoimmune diseases affecting the eyelids are pemphigus, discoid lupus erythematosus, systemic lupus erythematosus and bullous pemphigoid. Diagnosis requires biopsies for histopathology and immunofluorescence.

## Demodectic Mange

Younger dogs are especially prone to demodicid infections of the eyelids. A small area of hair loss usually occurs around the upper eyelid. Skin scrapings will reveal demodectic mites. Treatment for localized infections usually requires topical miticidal agents. Generalized demodicosis will require more potent miticidal treatment, and possibly antibiotic therapy. There are other ailments, such as allergic dermatitis and contact dermatitis.

# Anal Sac Ailments

Nobody really knows for certain what purpose the two anal sacs serve, but every dog's got them. The two sacs, located between the external and internal sphincter muscles on both side of the anus and including ducts that enter into the anal area, may be used to mark territory. Secretion usually occurs during defecation. Anal sac disease — *anal sacculitis* — is more common in smaller breeds of dogs, most typically in poodles, chihuahuas, Manchesters, spaniels and small mixed breeds. Large breeds are affected much less, although in their category the ailment is more common with the German shepherd and Doberman pinscher.

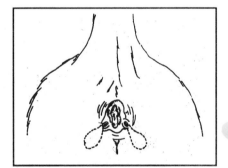

Figure 15.1 *Shown here is a diagrammatic representation of the anal sacs, their position and their duct openings.*

The normal anal sac secretion is a thick, straw-colored liquid with a very pungent odor. A dry pasty clay- to black-colored substance is usually an indicator of impactment, which means the glands are becoming all clogged up. A red- or green-colored liquid is a sign of infection. Anal sac abnormalities occur secondarily to infection or impaction. Symptoms usually include scooting, licking, obvious pain in the anal area, or abscessation with an open draining lesion.

The anal sacs can be "squeezed out" by laterally compressing on either side of the anus and anal sac area. Disposable gloves should be worn for this quick procedure. Impacted or infected anal sacs should have veterinary treatment. The veterinarian will first express (literally, squeeze out) the sac, then flush it with saline and antibiotic solutions, and possibly hot packs. Abscessation may need curettage, flushing and systemic antibiotics. Surgical excision of the anal sacs may be necessary for recurrent impaction, abscessation or fistulation. Excision results in a permanent cure.

# 16

# MISCELLANEOUS DISEASES

## ACQUIRED ALOPECIA

*By Dr. Al Becker, Northfield, Illinois*

One of the most perplexing and visibly distressing skin problems is *alopecia*, or hair loss. There are many types of alopecia, but in this chapter we will focus exclusively on those forms which are *acquired*. Most of the diseases that cause hair loss, based on clinical diagnoses, are of unknown origin. Some may be caused by genetics, breed disposition, history of physical injury or hair loss due to excessive grooming. All alopecia lesions should be scraped, cultured if possible, and biopsies performed. Remember that there are three stages of hair growth: *anagen* (growth), *telogen* (resting) and *catagen* (in between growth and rest). Each phase has different characteristics which can be visualized anatomically and explained functionally. (Many of these are explained in Chapter One.) Knowing what is normal can help us understand and identify abnormality.

### Problems that Plague Our Pets

Following is a list of various types of alopecia that afflict cats and dogs:

• **Pattern baldness** exists in the dachshund breed, but can be seen in Manchester terriers, miniature pinschers and the Chihuahua. There is currently no treatment for this condition.

• **Preauricular feline alopecia** is common and normal in cats. The temporal area between the eye and ear is involved. It is more commonly seen in short-haired cats, as the longer-coated animals tend to hide the alopecia.

•**Post-clipping alopecia** is seen mainly in sled dogs. Clipping causes an arrest in the catagen (in-between growth/rest) phase of hair growth. It is only temporary, and re-growth will occur after a hair growth cycle or two. That's why you should exercise great care before clipping sled dogs for any reason.

•**Post-rabies vaccine alopecia** appears mainly in toy and small breed dogs. The lesions appear two to three months after subcutaneous rabies vaccination, and are a result of a hypersensitivity reaction in the skin. Similar reactions, although transitory, occur with subcutaneous injections of steroids and occasionally penicillin.

•**Alopecia areata** is a non-inflammatory hair loss that is seen mainly in the head and neck area. It can occur in multicolored dogs, and involves hair loss in only one of the colors. This condition has been seen in Airedales and boxers in which hair loss is split along two sides of the pre-pubic area. It occurs mainly in late autumn and winter, and re-growth occurs by the summer. These dogs show no abnormalities in their thyroid and other hormonal functions. The condition is not inflammatory.

•**Pinnal alopecia** in dogs and cats is prevalent especially in dachshunds, Boston terriers, Chihuahuas, whippets, Italian greyhounds and Siamese cats. In the cat, the hair tends to regrow after several months. In the dog the tendency is for hair loss to begin after one year of age and to continue until total alopecia is reached at eight or nine years old. Some of the treatments that may help include thyroid therapy and the use of testosterone in male dogs. In the cocker spaniel, seborrhea of the ear margins can cause alopecia. Miniature poodles have a condition of periodic alopecia of the pinna (ear). Tufts of hair are suddenly lost from the pinna, resulting in bilateral alopecia. Hair regrowth occurs spontaneously within a few months.

•**Telogen effluvium** is a widespread alopecia resulting from metabolic stress, serious illness, high temperature, pregnancy, lactation or shock. It can also occur after surgery. There is a sudden hair loss (usually some weeks after the metabolic insult), followed by a re-growth some two or three months later as a new hair follicle cycle begins. Animals can also lose hair following the use of anti-cancer drugs, resulting in an interference of the anagen (hair growth) phase.

•**Canine traction alopecia** results from rubber bands and barrettes that are often placed on breeds such as the poodle, Maltese, Yorkshire terrier and shih-tzu. The decorative pieces create an actual traction on hair and skin, with no hope of re-growth in those areas of alopecia.

•**Scarring (cicatricial) alopecia** is a condition of permanent damage to the hair follicles. The causes may be physical or chemical, thermal, deep bacterial infections, neoplastic and auto-immune diseases. A good history and biopsy are essential in establishing this, as well as most alopecia conditions.

•**Feline endocrine alopecia** is a bilaterally symmetrical alopecia of cats, especially Siamese and Abyssinian breeds, involving the genital and perianal areas. It is not endocrine in origin, but is rather a psychogenic alopecia where the hair loss results from excessive grooming or chewing, often secretive. In order to clarify the diagnosis, the veterinarian must first rule out feline atopic disease, flea allergy and food allergy. The use of Elizabethan collars may be helpful in making a diagnosis, since hair growth will occur if the animals are not able to groom the sensitive areas. Various treatments have been used, all with some success, including L-thyroxine, male and female hormones, valium and phenobarbital.

Many other alopecic diseases are of hormonal origin (hypothyroidism, hyperadrenocorticism, hyper/hypoandrogenism and Sertoli cell tumor) and are discussed elsewhere in this book. The genetic alopecias (Blue and Fawn Doberman Syndrome) and follicular dysplasia also are discussed in other chapters.

As in all dermatological diseases, an animal with hair loss may have a myriad of diseases. The animal's age, breed, sex and clinical history, supportive diagnostic tests and response to therapy all will help lead the veterinarian to a conclusion as to what exactly is causing the hair loss.

# Psychogenic Dermatosis

By Dr. Steven A. Melman, Potomac, Maryland

The effect of the mind on dermatological — and other — health conditions is often overlooked by veterinary clinicians until all other diagnoses are eliminated. This is because psychogenic dermatoses and other disorders, such as those which cause itching, have many clinical signs in common. Veterinarians have identified a subset of diseases that seem to have a psychogenic component. They include lick granulomas, self-mutilation disorders, obsessive/compulsive disorders and psychogenic alopecia and dermatitis.

Psychogenic dermatosis always has a dermatologic as well as behavioral component. Since we know much more about the skin of domestic animals than we do about their mind, we start by taking a thorough history followed by an exhaustive clinical workup. When dermatologic causes have been eliminated, the search begins for a behavioral diagnosis. Historical questions may be personal. Has there been a change in the household? A child going off to college, a new baby, a breakup in a relationship, death of a family member or another pet, moving of furniture and changing residences have all been causes of psychogenic dermatosis cases suspected by the author. It seems that in our diagnostic efforts, we have resorted to classifying psychogenic dermatoses in terms of response to therapy. They are:

1) those that respond to behavioral drugs alone;

2) those that respond to a combination of drugs, including behavioral drugs; and

3) those that do not respond to therapy. Although a recent breakthrough in therapy gives cause for hope, it is thought that obsessive/compulsive disorders fit into the latter category.

Most research on how these disorders come about—their pathophysiology—involves the study of itching. The pathway is supposed to be as follows:

> *A stimulus (causing an itch) reaches a cell which releases a chemical which binds to another cell, and triggers a reaction which is transported by nerves to the spinal cord, which takes it to the brain, causing a response which is itching.*

There are various types of itch, including localized, spontaneous, pathologic and other forms. Itching may actually help relieve itself, although it is generally believed to be self-perpetuating. Itching is supposed to cause the release of endorphins, the body's natural pain killers. Itching is believed to increase in animals with behavioral problems, or those suffering from factors which might affect them. This *Gate Control Theory* is based on the premise that people who are under pressure are more likely to have a lower threshold for itching than those who are not. The following is a list of diseases which are believed to have at least a psychogenic component. They will briefly be described. The chapter will then discuss therapy, including some newer therapies.

## Lick Granulomas

Lick Granulomas (also known as acral lick dermatitis or ALD) are a raised, ulcerative, plaque which is commonly seen, most often on the dorsal aspect (front) of the front or hind legs. Most veterinarians seem to think they have a successful treatment plan ranging from cobra venom to intralesional injections of long-acting corticosteroids. Yet since the early days of veterinary practice, these cases have remained a challenge, known for their resistance to therapy. Often owners are resigned to the long-term presence of these lesions, which they believe the dog is obsessively and compulsively licking.

Some breeds seem to be over-represented. Large breeds such as golden retrievers and Labrador retrievers seem to be at risk, particularly if they become bored, as when they're left at home all day. Lick granulomas are usually deeply infected by the same bacteria, *Staphylococcus intermedius*, that causes other skin infections (see chapter 5 on Pyoderma). These infections are often complicated with other organisms. They are so deep that they may cause a proliferate in the underlying bone, in a reaction known as periosteal proliferation. It has been reported that some animals may have a sensory nerve deficit.

All animals need to be worked up for other causes. Allergy in particular may also be a complicator in ALD cases. One of the most common signs of allergy is foot-licking. The dog may also have a bone tumor or infection, ringworm, foreign body, demodex or an endocrine disorder such as hypothyroidism or hyperadrenocorticism. Treatment almost always involves long-term use of an antibiotic which kills the *S. intermedius*. My preference is cephalexin. Erythromycin can also be effective since it kills bacteria and also has an anti-inflammatory action. Trimethoprin-sulfa drugs — such as Bactrim, Ditrim or Tribrissen — are usually inadequate in treating these deep skin infections. Therapy should continue for at least three to four weeks beyond clinical cure. This often means giving antibiotics for three to six months.

Topical shampoo therapy should include the use of a benzoyl peroxide shampoo formulation, such as DermaPet Benzoyl Peroxide and Benzoyl Peroxide Plus. Mupirocin ointment can be applied topically since it penetrates skin well and is effective against *Staphylococcus*; however, it will be ineffective if the dog licks it off before the ointment has had adequate contact time. Using a tricyclic antidepressant such as Prozac (fluoxatime) or Anafranil (clomipramine) has been shown to help control the obsessive/compulsive urges of the affected animal. A study conducted with dogs, by a pioneer in researching human obsessive/compulsive disorders (OCD), showed promise. The author has been able to control numerous cases with Prozac and antibiotic therapy.

## Self-Mutilation

Self-mutilation disorders are not uncommon, although poorly understood and difficult to treat. Attention-seeking behavior, boredom and separation anxiety are all believed to be causes. A subset of people and animals are believed to have decreased sensitivity to pain. This is attributed to an abundance of endorphins (the body's natural pain killers), and to areas with a high level of receptors and thus a high resistance to pain. Boredom is thought to be an overused excuse for a cause. If the animal becomes occupied with activities in which he is interested, such as toys that play back, then the clinical signs of mutilation should disappear if the cause really was boredom. Animals that exhibit attention-seeking behavior, including tail chewing/chasing and limb-chewing, do this to get a response from the owner. This is frequently treated by training the owner not to respond, therefore failing to re-enforce the negative attention-seeking disorder. On the other hand, attention must be given to the affected pet, even if negative.

Separation anxiety is demonstrated by an animal that cannot be left alone. Often the animal will howl, growl, scratch, lick, chew, bite or mutilate itself when left alone. This is different from attention-seeking behavior, in which the animal may for example unroll a roll of toilet paper to get the owner's attention. Treatment in these cases often involves a combination of behavior modification and anti-anxiety drugs. Supplying toys that play back is often helpful. Although benzodiazepines are widely used to treat these cases, they should not be used, since they decrease the pet's ability to learn. Conversely, tri-cyclic anti-depressants such as Prozac should be acceptable, since they allow the pet to learn behavior modification.

## Obsessive/Compulsive Disorders (OCDs)

Behavior modification has no place in treating Obsessive/Compulsive Disorders (OCDs). In these cases, the behavior is ritualistic, and may or may not involve self-mutilation. Prozac and Anafranil, as mentioned above, have been very successful in treating human trichotillomania—an OCD in which a person pulls out his hair—as well as obsessive/compulsive hand-wringing or hand-washing. Treatment with this class of drugs often dooms humans and pets to lifelong therapy, since recurrence is common if the drug is removed. It is believed that many cases of ALD and attention-seeking disorders are OCDs.

## Feline Psychogenic Alopecia and Neurodermatitis

Feline Psychogenic Alopecia and Neurodermatitis are uncommon diseases of cats. They manifest as stubbled, broken-off hairs, often with a bilaterally symmetric distribution. Although the location varies, the affected area always appears well-delineated. The difference between the alopecic and neurodermatitic forms is that in the neurodermatitic form, the skin is also affected. Neurodermatitic lesions include excoriations and hemorrhagic (bloody) crusts. The most important diagnostic clue is the presence of hairs that are broken off. High-strung breeds like Siamese, Abyssinians and Burmese seem predisposed to this disease. Cats often will groom excessively when their owners are not present, leading to the term "closet-lickers." A thorough work-up is required, since no single reliable diagnostic test exists. The most common cause of itching in cats is believed to be flea allergy dermatitis, followed by food allergy and allergic inhalant dermatitis. Treatment is based on eliminating the underlying cause, frequently impossible.

## Therapy

There are a myriad of therapies available; none appears ultimately successful at curing psychogenic dermatoses. First I will discuss *inappropriate* treatments, notably physical restraints, surgery, amphetamines, topical therapy and tranquilizers. Although inappropriate treatments are usually ineffective by themselves, they may fit into an effective treatment plan. For example, while topical benzoyl peroxide and mupirocin ointment by themselves almost always fail in treating ALD, they can work as part of an overall treatment regimen. The key to successful treatment of ALD, OCD and mutilation disorders is to decrease the desire for focusing on the area which is affected.

Physical restraint devices like Elizabethan collars and bandaging may only increase the pet's desire to focus on the area. Nevertheless, these devices may be necessary in severe cases to temporarily alleviate severe self-trauma. Pets usually focus on an area above or below a bandage, even if it has a bitter taste. Topical treatments usually are licked off before they can be effective. Surgical removal may be necessary, but probably will not cure the problem; often the pet will just re-focus its attention on the remaining area. Amphetamine use should be restricted to treating hyperactive dogs, which are very rare. Tranquilizers do not produce typical behavior in the pet, and therefore can cloud and confuse a diagnostic work-up. Progestins like Ovaban, Depoprovera and Megace are excellent anti-itch medications which possess severe side-effects. These side-effects include testes enlargement, mammary gland hyperplasia, polyuria and polydipsia (drinking and urinating excessively), diabetes, bone marrow suppression, bladder abnormalities, alopecia and skin thinning.

Drugs considered appropriate include corticosteroids, narcotic antagonists, antihistamines and tricyclic antidepressants. As the above subjects are discussed, the recommended therapies will be briefly explained. Corticosteroids may cause severe side-effects (see Chapter 9 on corticosteroids). These drugs may themselves cause behavioral problems, including increased appetite, increased thirst, increased urination (including a change in housebreaking) and mood changes. Animals which already have an aggression problem while eating should be given these drugs with caution.

Narcotic antagonists include two drugs that can reverse the insensitivity to pain associated with mutilation or aberrant tail- chasing. They are Naltrexone, an injectable narcotic antagonist, and Talwin, a mixed narcotic agonist/antagonist. If the animal responds effectively to this therapy, then the location of the lesion is at the level of endorphin metabolism.

Atarax (hydroxyzine) is an antihistamine with a central depressive effect that has reduced itching in 20 to 50 percent of cases. It is available in oral, liquid or tablet form. Most experts agree that the trade-name drug should be used first to see if it is effective before resorting to generic derivatives, which may be of poorer quality.

Tricylcic antidepressants (TCAs) have been most helpful where the animal has a component of anxiety—be it separation, attention-seeking or an OCD. The author has found one TCA, Prozac, effective in treating atopic (allergic inhalant dermatitic) itches; possibly this allows pets to increase the threshold necessary to make them itch. Doxepin also has proven effective on occasion in the author's hands, as an antihistamine for itching cases that may be accompanied by urticaria (fluid filled bumps uncommonly seen in allergic animals).

Doxepin is 67 times more potent than Atarax (hydroxyxine) as a classical antihistamine, and 800 times more potent than Benadryl (diphenhydramine). In general, this class should not be used with MAO inhibitors, anticonvulsants (especially phenytoin/dilantin), steroids, antihistamines, aspirin or anticoagulants. Doxepin should not be used if the pet suffers from glaucoma or urinary retention.

The TCAs—including Anafranil (clomipramine), Elevil (amitriptyline) and Prozac (fluoxatime)—are contraindicated in cardiac cases. Reduced doses should be given in kidney and liver disease patients, since the drug is metabolized by the liver. TCAs also have been implicated in thyroid problems.

Side-effects of all TCAs include dry mouth and increased water consumption, with resultant excessive urination. Humans also have withdrawal side-effects — including anxiety piloerection, restlessness and diarrhea — although these are uncommon in domestic animals.

## Conclusion

Psychogenic dermatoses are a poorly understood group of diseases. It is believed that most are combined problems, although primary psychogenic dermatoses are evident in ALD, mutilation, feline traumatic alopecia and obsessive compulsive disorders. New therapeutic agents and treatment plans have given clinicians reason for optimism. However, the signs of pruritus (licking, biting, chewing, sucking and scratching) commonly seen in many disorders—most notably those of allergic origin—will remain difficult to distinguish as psychogenic in origin. They should therefore be considered non-psychogenic until other causes are eliminated.

# Feline Eosinophilic Granuloma Complex and Miliary Dermatitis

*By Dr. Steven A. Melman, Potomac, Maryland*

Eosinophilic granuloma, eosinophilic plaque and linear granuloma are a group of diseases affecting the skin and oral cavity of cats. Together, they comprise the *Eosinophilic Granuloma Complex* (EGC). The vast literature on this subject, instead of simplifying it, seems to justify the use of the term "complex." While EGC is often improperly used as a final diagnostic term, there are in fact many primary causes. It might be more accurate to call these clinical reaction patterns, which indicate a certain type of disease. Most frequently, cats have some sort of allergic reaction associated with EGC. This usually involved an allergy either to food, inhalants or insects. Although cats seem to be much less predisposed to bacterial infections than dogs are, bacteria appears to play a role occasionally, judging from the fact that some cases of EGC have responded to antibiotics. Recent studies have shown that some cats may have a hereditary predisposition to infection even when there is no clinical evidence of allergy.

*Miliary dermatitis* is believed to be the most typical reaction pattern of feline allergy. "Miliary" is merely a term describing a condition in which a cat has small papules and crusts accompanied by an inflammatory reaction.

*Feline symmetric hypotrichosis* is a disease in which cats manifest self-induced hair loss (alopecia) in a symmetric fashion. Again, the most common diagnosis would be allergy, followed closely by behavioral abnormalities. The most common misdiagnosis is feline endocrine alopecia, which most experts believe is very rare. The only way for a veterinarian to determine whether the hair would fall out on its own or is being actively licked out is to apply an Elizabethan collar. If the hair grows back, then the problem is either psychological or allergic. The next logical step would be to do an allergy work-up.

The *eosinophil* is believed to be the primary cell seen in allergic disorders of cats. It is the primary cell found both in tissue and in the circulation of EGC. In all species, it is believed to be involved in removing parasites, micro-organisms and complexes in the blood. The primary allergy cell — the mast cell — contains chemicals which it releases when contacted by an antigen which triggers it. These chemicals from the mast cell include one which calls eosinophils. Eosinophils also contain chemicals, two of which are the main cause of the clinical signs and pathological lesions seen in EGC.

Allergies can be caused by food, pollen or other environmental allergens and insects. Fleas are the most common cause of allergy in cats and probably the most common cause of disease in domestic animals. We now know that other insects—black flies and mosquitoes—are more common in causing EGC than most people originally thought. One investigator from Australia found insect protein in a piece of skin taken from an oral lesion from a cat with eosinophilic granuloma. Eosinophilic granulomas in humans, as described with typical biopsy findings, are most commonly a result of an insect bite.

# Clinical Signs

There are three types of EGC. It is common for more than one type to appear in the same cat, either simultaneously or over a longer period of time. They are:

### Eosinophilic ulcers

Also known as rodent ulcers and lip ulcers. They almost always occur in the upper lip, are not more likely to be found in any one breed, and are more commonly seen in females. They most often occur on the midline of the upper lip, but can also occur in the mouth and on the foot. These ulcers can progress to eat away a large amount of tissue, causing the cat to either look like a rat or look as though it has been bitten by one. They usually are not painful and do not itch.

### Eosinophilic plaques

Eosinophilic plaques almost always itch severely. Itching almost always precedes the appearance of the lesions. They appear first as papules, and progress into plaques which often ulcerate. These typically appear on the abdomen and flank, and occur in younger cats.

### Linear granulomas

Also known as eosinophilic/collagenolytic granulomas or true granulomas. These also occur most commonly in young cats, especially females. The classical lesion is located on the back of the hind legs and is a raised, linear (straight line) granuloma progressing up the leg. However, it also has been identified in the mouth, on the bridge of the nose, on the ear, and on the footpad and paws. The differential diagnosis includes tumors, lesions caused by an organism (bacterial or fungal) or foreign bodies. Occasionally, chronic lesions such as plaques can be associated with feline leukemia virus, or feline immunodeficiency virus.

# Diagnosis

Careful history and physical examinations are required. A complete blood count along with a biopsy will reveal findings to the trained veterinarian. Oddly enough, the presence of an increase in the eosinophil count in tissue and/or the circulation is usually seen only in eosinophilic plaque. A proper allergy work-up is important, including tests for food, insect and inhalant allergy. If there is a bacterial infection, it should require only topical therapy or perhaps properly selected systemic antibiotic as well. Treatment will depend on the diagnosis. If the cause is allergy, then avoidance works best. However, while one can avoid food and perhaps certain insects, some environmental allergens may require an allergy vaccine for hypo-sensitization.

### Glucocorticoids

Glucocorticoids seem to be the treatment of choice, with best results occurring after using Depomedrol (methylprednisolone acetate). The pet owner should be aware that this drug is long-lasting and can suppress not only the immune response that causes the problem but also the one which might protect the cat at the same time. Nevertheless, even the best practitioners will use two to three injections back-to-back at two-week intervals. Topical glucocorticoids do not work in the cat, since the product is usually licked off. What effect they might have on a cat with an Elizabethan collar needs to be properly assessed.

Ovaban (megestrol acetate) has been used as a treatment. Besides the fact that it is not licensed for use in cats, it should not be used because it causes many side-effects. Mammary gland lesions, known as fibradenomateous hyperplasia, may not disappear simply because the drug is continued. Similarly, using this drug may cause diabetes mellitus. Behavioral abnormalities, weight gain and lethargy are other common side-effects. Perhaps the most serious complication is the suppression of the adrenal gland, which occurs at even low doses and persists for weeks. Other methods of treatment include excisional surgery, cryosurgery, radiation and lasers. Of these, the most practical to the author seems to be carbon dioxide laser therapy which, although only reported in one study, seems to have a favorable response rate.

I look forward to someday re-naming this syndrome *Eosinophilic Granuloma simplex*. But for the time being, many of these cases seem to defy a logical work-up, and normal clinical treatment remains as mysterious as most felines are themselves.

# Shar-Pei Problems

*By Dr. Steven A. Melman, Potomac, Maryland*

I often wonder, when I see a Shar-Pei in the waiting room of my clinic, whether the pet owner was warned before shelling out any money that he was purchasing a breed which is known in some circles as a "veterinary dermatologist's delight." The only problem is, despite a very extensive and often expensive work-up, the end result is not always a healthy dog. This breed is fraught with skin conditions. Of all the breeds, the Shar-Pei is reported to have the highest incidence of allergic disorders, demodex, pyoderma, otitis externa and hypothyroidism. It also appears they are unique in their predisposition to Immunoglobulin A deficiency (the surface surveillance immunoglobulin) and to cutaneous mucinosis, an otherwise uncommon ailment. Of course, Shar-Pei breeders should be advised that not every line is always affected. I have been assured that healthy Shar-Pei do exist; in fact, I've even seen some of them. By and large, Shar-Pei breeders and owners are a responsible and likable lot. Let's look at some of the more common dermatological problems that plague those wrinkled dogs.

## Allergic Diseases

Various studies have shown that up to 67.2 percent of Shar-Pei with skin diseases are thought to have an allergy of some sort. That makes it the breed with the *highest relative risk for allergy*. Of the 67.2 percent of ailing Shar-Pei with allergy, almost half have a pyoderma. Food allergy was seen in about 15 percent; flea allergy (which is the most common allergic disease) was only present about 20 percent of the time. Contact allergy, which the author rarely diagnoses, has been seen concurrently with atopy and food allergy.

*Atopy* is the most common disease, and (as described in the Chapter 8) is usually associated with itching. *Otitis Externa* is a common complication of atopy. It can be seen without allergy, thanks largely to the Shar-Pei's unusual ear shape — which is naturally constricted (stenotic). It is not unusual to see chronic cases of both allergy and otitis (See Chapters 8 and 14). Although most breeds do not show clinical signs of allergy until after one year of age, more than 80 percent of Shar-Pei will show signs of allergy long before their first birthday. Not much to celebrate when you're a young Shar-Pei!

*Food allergy* (See Chapter 8, page 119) may be difficult to discern from atopy. Therefore, all Shar-Pei with signs of allergy should undergo a vigorous food elimination diet. I usually recommend a hypoallergenic diet in all my allergy cases, for this limits the possibility of a reduced itch-threshold. A bit of explanation is needed here by way of example: A dog may be sensitive to eggs, but not enough to cause serious itchiness. It has a relatively "high" threshold to this offending substance. However, the same dog may also be hypersensitive to ragweed. When ragweed season hits with a fury, the poor dog's ability to tolerate beef declines, and what was once an "egg sensitivity" now becomes a serious hypersensitivity. The result is an animal that now suffers from both ragweed and eggs. To veterinarians, this phenomenon is known as "summation of effect." Quite often, the Shar-Pei will develop multiple types of allergy.

## Folliculitis

One of the most common skin problems seen in veterinary dermatology, folliculitis is almost always caused by the *Staphylococcus intermedius* bacteria (See Chapter 5 on Pyoderma). The Shar-Pei shows clinical signs of skin infection (folliculitis) different from most breeds. Whereas most breeds develop pustules and the round, scaly epidermal collarettes, the Shar-Pei ends up looking like a band of moths have attacked it. This is typically known as "moth-eaten alopecia (hair loss)." The pyoderma affecting Shar-Pei is almost always secondary to an allergy of some type, but can be a direct result of IgA deficiency (described later). The propensity of this breed to have excessive skin folds has opened them up to skin-fold infections. Treatment almost always includes frequent bathing with benzoyl peroxide preparations. Occasionally, systemic antibiotics are necessary.

## IgA Deficiency

In humans, the most common immunoglobulin deficiency is IgA Deficiency. Don't feel left out, because German shepherds and beagles also suffer from deficiencies of IgA, the surface surveillance immunoglobulin. Well, when it comes to Shar-Pei, such deficiencies are, it seems, to be expected. In fact, I have seen a case (and heard of others) in which a dog had no measurable IgA at all! Such individuals have been virtually doomed to an existence of recurrent infection. It appears that IgA may leave an animal vulnerable to invasion by antigens. Immunoglobulin E (the allergy immunoglobulin) appears to be designed for a perfect match with some of these antigens. Without them, the dog is doomed to a life of itching and atopy or food allergy.

## Hypothyroidism

Only about 3.4 percent of a series of Shar-Pei with skin disease were reported to have hyperthyroidism. Although this is a relatively high percentage for many other breeds, it does not approach the level of the Doberman or other high-risk breeds.

## Demodex

*The Shar-Pei has the highest relative risk factor of any other breed when it comes to demodex.* It is not usually inflamed unless there is an associated folliculitis. Every Shar-Pei with a skin disease should have a deep and thorough skin scraping. Although *Demodex* is usually an easy mite to scrape, a negative skin scraping in this breed should not rule out demodex, as is commonly the case in other breeds. The good news is that they often regress and respond quite well to standard amitraz (Mitaban) therapy, along with treatment for associated clinical signs such as folliculitis.

## Idiopathic Mucinosis

The genetic selection for wrinkled skin seems to have predisposed even normal Shar-Pei to idiopathic (cause unknown) *mucinosis*, which leaves the dogs vulnerable to excessive mucin production. Mucin is normally found in small quantities in the dermis, and is responsible for normal structure, support, nutrition and mineral balance. It can be show up as either thickened skin or with intradermal vesicles. These vesicles can be ruptured easily by a pin to exude a thick, clear, sticky fluid. *Hypothyroidism* does not appear to be related. It usually occurs in the first year of life; many cases normally are outgrown by two to five years. For those who prefer treatment, corticosteroids are the drug of choice. However, these drugs are also overused in the treatment of many Shar-Pei itching disorders. Unfortunately, for those who especially enjoy the many folds of skin, corticosteroids may deflate the Shar-Pei by decreasing skin wrinkling and skin thickness.

# Diseases of
# West Highland White Terriers

*By Dr. Margreet W. Vroom, Oisterwijk, The Netherlands*

I s it necessary to write a chapter on just West Highland white terriers? Do all Westies have skin problems? In truth, the situation is really not that bad, but Westies can have skin disorders which may be difficult to treat. If you own a Westie, you would be smart to know all these problems so that if your pet does show signs of trouble, you can start treatment early on.

## Seborrhea

Almost every dog with a skin problem will show signs of secondary seborrhea. But in those instances when seborrhea develops on its own, independent of any other dermatological problem, then you are dealing with a primary seborrhea. Seborrhea is a combination of a hyperkeratosis (excessive scale production) and abnormal sebaceous gland funtion. (See Chapters 4 and 11.) Westies can be prone to a seborrhea oleosa, which normally occurs in the axilla and groin, generalized or just on the back. This fatty seborrhea can cause itch (pruritus), as well as a bacterial inflammation (See Chapter 5) or yeast (See Chapter 6) infection. Many Westies with seborrhea develop a hyperpigmentation (black skin) with alopecia (hairlessness) and hyperkeratosis (thick skin).

Secondary pyoderma (bacterial inflammation) may contribute to the severity of this condition. An ear inflammation (otitis externa) can occur. The dogs always scratch, bite and chew. The best thing you can do is look for a *primary* cause of the seborrhea. This chapter will discuss these causes, while the treatment of a seborrhea is left to a more complete discussion in Chapter 11.

As far as my dogs are concerned, they get shampooed twice a week. It is important to use a shampoo containing benzoyl peroxide (such as Mycodex BP or DermaPet Benzoyl Peroxide Plus) when the skin is inflamed. Look for papules and pustules. In cases where there is greasy skin, a tar shampoo may be helpful, with benzoyl peroxide as an alternative. But be careful with these ingredients, which can be irritating. Often when these cases become controlled, a milder shampoo, with just sulfur and salicylic acid, such as DermaPet Seborrheic shampoo, can be used for maintenance (See Chapter 4).

## Food Allergy

In a retrospective study I performed on 45 Westies in the Netherlands, I found 11 Westies (24 percent) with a food allergy. This is a very high percentage. The clinical signs first made their appearance in dogs between four and 18 months of age. All dogs had pruritus and developed a pyoderma, while five just chewed on their front feet. Some dogs showed a generalized seborrhea with pyoderma, and others had seborrhea only on the back. Many dogs had concomitant *otitis externa*. Diagnosis was made by feeding these dogs a home cooked hypoallergenic diet consisting of lamb or turkey with rice and some green vegetables. (Without any fiber in the diet, a dog can get diarrhea.) The duration of the diet varied from three weeks to three months.

The average time before the skin returned to normal was almost eight weeks, which says that you need a lot of time and patience before you can expect to see results. After the skin was back to normal, the affected dogs were challenged with the original food, just to see if the skin problems will re-occur. This is absolutely necessary. You may discover, for example, that the food allergy was caused by dog biscuits. Then you can let your dog eat its normal food without restriction. If, on the other hand, you discover the dog's normal kibble is the offending allergen (substance that can cause allergy), a lifelong altered diet will be necessary: A hypoallergenic diet with a vitamin and mineral supplementation, for instance, or a commercial hypoallergenic dog food.

You've got to stick to the special diet very strictly, and no cheating! Even one piece of cheese in a week can ruin the entire diet. If you can discover the offending agent (the ingredient that is causing the allergic reaction), the prognosis will be excellent. Meanwhile, you must continue to treat any secondary bacterial inflammations and secondary yeast infections (See Chapters 4 and 6).

## Atopy

Of the 45 Westies I mentioned above, six appeared to have atopy. The most important clinical signs (which began between five months and three years of age) were pruritus, pyoderma and seborrhea. It was impossible to differentiate a dog with atopy from a dog with a food allergy without further investigation. The age of onset and the clinical signs can be identical. The diagnosis of atopy was made after a six-week hypoallergenic diet was unsuccesful and an intradermal skin test came back positive (See Chapter 8).

# Demodex

Of the 45 Westies, three appeared to have demodicosis, a mite-related disease (See Chapter 7). A primary immunosuppressive disorder allows the mite to multiply. In all three demodex cases, primary causes were discovered: atopy, food allergy and flea allergy. Other possibilities you can't ignore may be diabetes mellitus, kidney- and liver-functioning, stress, viral infections, etc. The typical treatment for demodex is to clip the entire dog. Every other day we dip our Westies with amitraz (Taktic) in a solution of 1 to 100, a treatment which is not approved in the United States. However, the amitraz liquid concentrate Mitaban is approved by the U.S. Food and Drug Administration for use in a two-week interval. The first treatment schedule has better results.

The unfortunate side-effects of amitraz include nausea, dizziness, diarrhea and erythema of the skin. Dogs which have not been clipped develop more toxic side-effects. The owner has to perform the treatment outside, wear plastic gloves and be carefull not to splash the solution in his or her face. The eyes of the dog are protected by applying vitamin A drops before the dipping. Pregnant women are warned not to perform the treatment. The treatment may last from six weeks to three months. When the disease is very difficult to cure, a primary cause is overlooked. This is easy to write down but sometimes difficult to prove. Prognosis varies from good to poor, depending of the primary cause.

# Malassezia Pachydermatis

This is a normal yeast which makes its home on the skin (See Chapter 6). However, when the normal condition of the skin changes, the yeast can multiply to unhealthy levels. The yeast loves a greasy skin. Does the yeast create a greasy skin for itself? We don't know. What we do know is that many Westies with fatty seborrhea often have an abundance of yeast organisms on their skin. Of the 45 Westies in my study, three needed treatment for the yeast. Only one was cured, while the two others experienced a temporary improvement. In other Westies I found yeast organisms as a secondary disorder, which I didn't treat. The primary problems these dogs had included food allergies. When the diet was altered, the skin cleared up and the yeast was gone.

The skin of a Westie with yeast infection is hyperpigmentated, hyperkeratotic, and smells quite bad. The skin feels greasy. The yeast may be limited to the axilla or interdigital area, but it can also be generalized or just in the ears. The dogs are pruritic. Treatment consists of shampooing the dog twice weekly with a benzoyl peroxide shampoo. The shampoo needs to be combined with a rinse of Nizoral (ketoconazole) every week. Another possibility is oral treatment. Ketoconazole tablets (Nizoral,

Janssen Pharm.) are useful. This medication can cause liver problems, vomiting, signs of malaise and abortion (it is teratogenic). Fortunately, most side-effects will never occur. I advise owners to give the medication with some food.

## Epidermal Dysplasia

This disorder causes extremely abnormal keratinization. Because it has only been found in the Westie, and because it starts at a very young age, it is likely that Epidermal Dysplasia is an inherited illness. The dogs first develop erythema (redness) of the skin, and there is pruritus as well. The hyperkeratosis develops very soon. Within one year of age, the dog is hyperpigmentated, alopecic and has a greasy seborrhea. It looks like an armadillo. Yeast infection is often found. A skin biopsy is necessary for a proper diagnosis. Also be careful to check for food allergy, primary seborrhea, atopy, yeast infections and scabies. Tragically, this illness is nonresponsive to treatment. Antibiotics, synthetic vitamin retinoids, corticosteroids, shampoos, essential fatty acids and vitamin E have been tried, without success. Because the dogs are very pruritic and no treatment will have any effect, the dogs are euthanized at a young age.

## Response to Essential Fatty Acids

The role of essential fatty acids in veterinary medicine is quite new, with new findings being published every year. These fatty acids have antipruritic effects, and can influence the amount of seborrhea. The greatest advantage is the lack of side-effects. In Westies, essential fatty acids can reduce the amount of pruritus and decrease the seborrhea. Patients with a food allergy or atopy can also benefit from this product. In my study of 45 Westies, two responded very well on essential fatty acids. In one dog the diagnosis was primary seborrhea and one was atopic. Both had no more skin problems after using the fatty acids during four weeks. Lifelong treatment may be necessary, although it is possible to reduce the dosage.

## Conclusion

If you own a Westie, you should examine your dog every day for potential skin problems. All of those skin diseases mentioned in this chapter must be identified and treated early, before a small problem develops into a big disaster. Eight of the 45 Westies I studied had to be euthanized. Their owners waited two to five years before taking their dogs to a veterinary dermatologist, and many owners were frustrated and unwilling to start all over again. Play it safe, and prevent problems before they arise. Westies need a thorough examination from the first signs of a skin ailment.

# 17

# NATURAL THERAPIES

*By Dr. Lowell Ackerman, Payson, Arizona*

Natural therapy is nothing new. After all, many of the most popular drugs used today were originally isolated from nature. For example, we often forget that aspirin (acetylsalicylic acid) was originally derived from the bark of willow trees, or that the digitalis used by heart patients actually comes from the foxglove plant. So there is obvious confusion when people talk about "natural remedies." Unfortunately, too many people go to extremes, and mere mention of a natural therapy brings to mind either miracle cures or quackery. Natural therapy is neither.

Conspiracy theories and anti-institution prejudices do not play a role in this chapter on natural therapies for skin disorders. The medical community is not on trial for converting plant-derived substances into laboratory produced "lookalikes," because there is a definite need for this conversion. The most obvious advantage is that conventional medicines are easier to study, because we know exactly how much of each ingredient has gone into their production. If problems occur in their later use, we can more easily determine what medicinal ingredient is at fault. This is often impossible with natural preparations, since actual concentrations of active ingredients may vary considerably between plants, or even between leaves on the same plant.

Then again, there are some natural remedies which cannot be distilled into one active ingredient. Take garlic, for example. It has been credited with many healing attributes, yet no one ingredient has been pinpointed for these benefits. Perhaps it is the allicin, the germanium, the allyl disulfides, the volatile oils or a combination of them all. Until conventional medicine isolates and purifies the exact beneficial ingredients in garlic, the bulb will remain under the category of natural remedy.

With that understanding in place, we can move on to explore some of the natural products that may play a role in treating disease and keeping pets healthy. We'll examine aloe vera, bioflavonoids, Brewer's yeast, bromelin, coenzyme Q, digestive enzymes, dimethylglycine, echinacea, garlic and ho-meopathic remedies. These natural products are generally regarded as safe, but it is important to realize that few studies have looked at their potential adverse effects on dogs or cats. Therefore, they must be used at the owner's risk and discretion.

## Aloe Vera

There are over 200 species worldwide of the "healing plant," aloe vera, from which this remedy is derived. For over a thousand years, aloe vera has been advocated as a natural treatment for cuts, burns and other skin problems. There are also those who advocate its being taken internally by patients with digestive problems, arthritis and allergies. Scientific study has indeed confirmed that aloe vera increased the rate of healing of burns and cuts, but fewer studies have been performed to show the merit of internal use. Because aloe vera contains such a hodgepodge of alkaloids, saponins, glycoproteins and terpenoids, is has been difficult to determine the most active ingredients.

For pets with arthritis, digestive problems and allergies, aloe vera may be useful. But positive clinical trials are few and far between. In a very limited study of 10 allergic dogs, none benefitted from taking aloe vera internally. However, the plant makes an excellent topical remedy for cuts, burns and inflamed skin. Recently, a complex carbohydrate derived from aloe called acemannan has proven to be a potent stimulator of the immune system. Research to date has shown that acemannan stimulates the release of interleukin-1 and tumor necrosis factor — two products of the immune system that help defend against infections and cancers.

Acemannan has been used experimentally in the treatment of infectious diseases, immunologic diseases, periodontal disease and some cancers. Recently, it has been licensed as a stimulant of the immune system for the treatment of a malignant cancer (fibrosarcoma) in dogs and cats. Acemannan appears to be an extremely safe derivative of aloe, and ongoing research may uncover many more positive applications.

## Bioflavonoids

Bioflavonoids have many similarities to vitamins, and are even sometimes referred to as "vitamin P." But they are not vitamins. Rather, they are polyphe-nolic plant compounds. Most bioflavonoids are derived from citrus fruits, from the white material just beneath the peel. An exception is the bioflavonoid quercitin, which is found in blue-green algae. The main action of bioflavonoids is to reduce inflammation, and there are several studies that show them to be beneficial in treating allergies. In fact, a synthetic flavonoid (Cromolyn™) is licensed for the treatment of asthma and allergies in humans.

Bioflavonoids stabilize small blood vessels and make them less permeable so they don't "leak." (That is why they were originally referred to as vitamin P.) This, in turn, stabilizes the mast cells and basophils that release histamine and cause allergic reactions. In this way, bioflavonoids provide the same effects as antihistamines. In both humans and dogs, the bioflavonoids quercitin and catechin appear to be the most effective in treating allergies and asthma. However, bioflavonoids act most effectively in combination with vitamin C. Health food stores usually carry natural allergy relief formulations based on bioflavonoids and vitamin C. Most are quite safe for use in pets and people.

## Brewer's Yeast

Brewer's yeast has been advocated not only as a nutritional supplement, but as a safeguard against fleas. As a nutritional supplement, it contains high levels of the amino acids lysine, tryptophan and threonine. It is also rich in B vitamins, except for cyanocobalamin ($B^{12}$). It is also deficient in the important sulfur-containing amino acids methionine and cystine. Since brewer's yeast is also high in phosphorus, large amounts should not be given to growing pups or elderly animals. The high phosphorus content could interfere with the use of calcium in bone development in young animals, while older pets could develop bad kidneys from too much phosphorus. Brewer's yeast should also be used cautiously in dogs with recurrent yeast infections, since sensitivity (allergy) could become a problem. Claims of brewer's yeast as an effective flea control agent have never stood up to scientific scrutiny, with repeated studies unable to prove that brewer's yeast protects pets against fleas. Still, some pet owners continue to stand behind brewer's yeast when fighting flea infestation.

## Bromelin

Originally isolated as a protein-breaking enzyme found in pineapple, bromelin was later shown to have anti-inflammatory properties. It is suspected that bromelin works by inhibiting the creating of certain inflammation-causing substances (prostaglandins) as they occur in the body. This is similar to the effects of aspirin, and yet bromelin does not interfere with blood clotting the way aspirin does. Because of its anti-inflammatory properties, bromelin has also been used to treat skin infections, allergies and burns. It may also be helpful following trauma or surgery. Too much remains unknown to allow comment on other potential benefits, but improvement was observed in dogs with arthritis. It is likely that the same mechanism that helps relieve the symptoms of allergy can also reduce the inflammation seen in sore, aching joints.

Bromelin is very safe, but it may cause digestive upsets in some dogs and cats. This enzyme supplement is available from most health food stores, and is also found in Prozyme, an enzyme supplement formulated for pets.

## Coenzyme Q

Here is an interesting nutrient that doesn't fit neatly into any category. Coenzyme Q resembles a vitamin, but it is not a vitamin. To complicate matters further, it is a coenzyme rather than an enzyme. It is often referred to as ubiquinone because it occurs everywhere that life is found. Chemically, as a quinone it is in the same family as vitamin K[1]. Coenzyme Q is found in every food source that has ever "breathed," including all plants, animals and microbes. However, the form of coenzyme Q that is needed by animals and humans comes only from vertebrate sources. This form is known as coenzyme $Q^{10}$.

Cells require coenzyme Q for energy production, and as an antioxidant. Most research has concentrated on its role in heart disease and high blood pressure. In these cases it appears to be effective for treatment of cardiomyopathy, as well as having some stabilizing role in heart rhythm. Humans suffering from angina, high blood pressure and even periodontal disease have benefitted from coenzyme Q supplementation, researchers found. Because of its role in supporting the immune system, coenzyme Q may be useful in treating dogs and cats plagued by allergies, recurrent infections or immunodeficiency syndromes. It appears to be an extremely safe nutrient. For the most benefit, supplements used should contain coenzyme $Q^{10}$, the most active form of the nutrient.

## Digestive Enzymes

Digestive enzyme preparations are commercially available for dogs and cats, including digestive enzyme products derived from either animal pancreases or plants. The pancreatic enzyme preparations often have three major digestive enzymes: *protease, amylase* and *lipase.*

- Protease (such as trypsin and chymotrypsin) breaks down dietary protein.

- Amylase digests sugars and starches.

- Lipase breaks down dietary fats.

- The plant-derived enzymes (such as Prozyme™) also digest cellulose, or dietary fiber. These enzymes are necessary so that food can be digested and later absorbed from the intestines.

Pancreatic enzymes may be prescribed by veterinarians when dogs have diseases that render the pancreas unable to produce its own enzymes. This is a condition referred to as pancreatic insufficiency. On the other hand, plant-derived enzymes such as Prozyme™ can be given to dogs and cats in an effort to maximize their ability to use all the nutrients they eat. An animal doesn't necessarily need to be "ill" in order to benefit from the maximum absorption of dietary nutrients.

Preliminary studies indicate that dogs and cats given Prozyme™ significantly increase their blood levels of zinc and selenium. There are also increases in blood pyridoxine (vitamin B⁶) and in the total digestibility of the diet. Additional studies are currently underway. Owners report many improvements from supplementation with these plant-based digestive enzymes, but these claims are only now being investigated.

It is presumed that many animals may have borderline levels of their own enzymes, and may not be able to make full use of what they're eating. The result is a relative vitamin and mineral imbalance, despite eating a good diet. Also, there is at least some circumstantial evidence that marginal pancreatic enzyme deficiencies might allow sufficient protein remnants to sensitize the intestinal lining, increasing susceptibility to food allergies or intolerances. At this point, there are more questions than answers.

Plant-based enzyme supplements such as Prozyme™ appear to be very safe and may be useful supplements for a variety of different situations — such as for elderly animals or those pets with digestive problems. Use of these supplements for skin problems are currently being studied. Theoretically, dogs with hair loss or poor hair growth may find some improvement with these therapies, since hair growth is a major nutritional drain on the body.

Most enzyme supplements are designed to be applied to the food before it is eaten, not given directly to the dog. The supplement should be applied to the food for several minutes before feeding, giving the enzymes an opportunity to break down the proteins, carbohydrates and fats before the food is consumed.

## Dimethyl Glycine

Originally called vitamin B¹⁵ or pangamic acid, dimethyl glycine (N,N-dimethylglycine) is not a vitamin at all. It is actually a tertiary amino acid.

Dimethyl glycine is not considered essential for dogs or cats, and, in fact, it has received very little attention from the pet food industry. The amino acid is present, in minute quantities, in sunflower seeds, brewer's yeast, rice bran, wheat bran, whole grain cereals, oat grits, corn grits, pumpkin seeds, sesame seeds, wheat germ and liver.

Dimethyl glycine is looked upon as an "enhancer" used to improve the functioning of the immune and cardiovascular systems. Because it appears to help oxygen uptake as well as stimulate response, dimethyl glycine may also have a place in the treatment of pets with immune deficits or with heart disease. Competing dogs may also benefit from the nutrient's enhancement of athletic performance. Supplementation with dimethyl glycine appears to be extremely safe, and the product is available in health food stores.

## Echinacea

The roots and leaves of the *Echinacea angustifolia* plant contain a variety of different ingredients, including betaine, echinacen, fatty acids and polysaccharides. Studies have shown that this herb increases the body's immune response against a variety of viruses and bacteria. Echinacea has been scientifically shown to increase levels of interferon (an immunologic fighter of viruses and cancers) in the body, as well as properdin, a protein that destroys bacteria and neutralizes viruses.

Research has also found that a compound called echinacen B can also inhibit inflammation in the body, especially that caused by hyaluronidase. This might make echinacea supplementation helpful when treating skin problems or even ailments of the joints. Echinacea can be used when a natural stimulant is needed to give the immune system a boost. A polysaccharide (sugar) portion of the echinacea extract appears to be the powerhouse behind this phenomenon. This can be useful when, for example, you have a pet that seems to constantly develop infections. However, because alcohol tinctures destroy the polysaccharide portion of the echinacea extract, freeze-dried preparations are preferable when the immune-stimulating qualities are called for. Echinacea capsules can be purchased from health food outlets. But be aware that although echinacea is extremely safe, it should only be used periodically — giving the immune system a chance to respond on its own.

## Garlic

Probably the most-prescribed herbal remedy, garlic acts as a natural antibiotic, immune stimulant, regulator of digestion and detoxifier. Contained within the garlic bulb are numerous chemicals, including unsaturated aldehydes, volatile oils, vitamins and minerals. In many clinical trials, garlic has been proven beneficial, but nobody knows exactly what ingredients in the herb are responsible for this.

Much research has focused on allicin and the allyl disulfides, but they only account for part of the picture. Research with humans suggests that garlic might lower cholesterol and triglycerides, as well as blocking the ability of cancer-causing chemicals (carcinogens) to turn normal cells into cancerous ones. Additional studies have proven helpful in stimulating various immunologic factors and protecting cells against damage from free radicals.

Garlic has been recommended for pets with flea problems, but there is little scientific evidence to back up this contention. Its best use is for pets with immune problems, digestive upsets or recurrent infections. Newer versions even lack the odor which has plagued garlic for centuries. In clinical trials performed at Chinese medical institutions, garlic was found to be as effective in the treatment of some fungal infections as conventional prescription drugs.

## Homeopathic Remedies

Eighteenth century German physician Samuel Hahnemann developed the medical treatment we now know as *homeopathy*. Hahnemann devised his "law of similitudes" in which patients were treated with medications that caused side-effects similar to the symptoms of the illness. In other words, vomiting patients were given extracts that would usually cause vomiting. He worked by trial and error, comparing the ills of his patients with the direct and indirect effects of various substances and with their capacity to produce or cure the illness concerned. This principle that "like is cured by like" separates homeopathy from every other type of therapeutic treatment.

Conventional (allopathic) medicine tends to look at treatment in dose-related fashion. That generally translates to mean that larger doses exert more effect on a patient. But homeopathy works in the opposite direction: The more serious the illness, the smaller the dose of therapy prescribed. Homeopathic practitioners prepare sequential dilutions of extracts called potentiation, and the final product may end up containing no measurable amount of the original extract. These potencies are a measure of the relative dilution of the concentrated drug, and they are denoted by a number which follows the name of the drug itself.

For example, with Arnica 6x or Sulfur 3x, the higher the number the greater the dilution. It is not unusual that the original extract be diluted over a million times in homeopathic remedies. In these examples, the sulfur 3x dilutes the original potency one thousand times ($10^3$), while the arnica 6x is diluted a million times ($10^6$). How these remedies might work at such extreme dilutions cannot be explained by contemporary modern science, and is a bone of contention between conventional physicians and homeopathic practitioners.

Today there are over 2,000 homeopathic remedies available, with about 60 percent derived from plant sources. The rest are mineral compounds or animal-derived products. Homeopathy is built around observations of individuals, and therefore there are no large-scale clinical trials proving this method's effectiveness. Most of the conventional medical establishment contends there is no scientific evidence to support homeopathy, but its proponents are equally positive that it works.

# 18

# TUMORS
# OF THE SKIN

*By Maj. Bruce H. Williams, Washington, D.C.*

The skin is the largest organ of the body. As such, it generates the largest numbers of tumors of any organ system. Before we discuss the different types of tumors encountered in the skin, it is important to define a few terms that will help you understand more about skin tumors. A *neoplasm* is the uncontrolled growth of a certain group of cells. It is distinguished by the type of cell it is made of; i.e., neoplasms of epithelial cells, or cells that line sweat glands, or cells that line hair follicles. Each type of neoplasm has its own individual *behavior*, such as rate of growth, and potential for *metastasis*, or spread to internal organs. A *veterinary pathologist* who is a specialist in the study of tumors can often make generalizations about the behavior of a neoplasm: most epithelial tumors tend to act a certain way, while most sweat gland tumors act in a different way, and so on. After graduation, *veterinary pathologists* undergo three to five years of additional training into the causes of animal diseases. They learn to diagnose diseases by the characteristic changes they see in the tissues of animals, either by visual inspection of the whole animal or with a microscope. In addition, *board-certified veterinary pathologists* must pass a rigorous certifying examination.

A *tumor* is a swelling of any sort. It may be due to a bee sting, a localized infection or a neoplasm. In the medical field, however, the word *tumor* is often used synonymously with *neoplasm*, and will be used in this fashion for the remainder of this chapter.

Neoplasms are often classified either *benign* or *malignant*. *Benign* neoplasms are generally more slow-growing and tend to expand in a nodular fashion, compressing the tissue around it. While growth of this type may be life-threatening in certain organs, such as in the brain or the lungs, it is rarely so in the skin. The vast majority of cutaneous neoplasms in dogs are benign. *Malignant* tumors, on the other hand, grow rapidly and invade surrounding tissues. They destroy and replace the adjacent structures of the skin. Malignant tumors cause greater damage than benign ones because they rapidly invade and replace healthy adjacent skin, and may metastasize. Not only do malignant tumors destroy the skin's protective function, but after metastasizing through blood and lymph vessels, they may destroy internal organs. Additionally, malignant tumors arising in other organs in the body may metastasize to the skin, where they may be diagnosed first.

When evaluating the benign or malignant nature of neoplasms, the pathologist will often give a *prognosis*, or a long-term forecast for the animal's health. Once removed, benign tumors generally carry a *good* prognosis, which means that the animal will most likely have no further ill effects. A *guarded* prognosis may be used when a malignant tumor is seen. Even though this tumor may be completely removed, metastasis may already have occurred prior to surgery. A small number of these cases have subsequent health problems as a result of the neoplasm, and may result in the death of this animal. A *poor* or *grave* prognosis is used when the neoplasm behaves in an aggressive fashion and has metastasized to internal organs. Luckily, tumors which carry a poor prognosis are rarely encountered in the skin.

## Causes of Skin Neoplasms

Neoplastic cell growth may be triggered by a number of compounds or substances. In human skin, the most widely known trigger is *ultraviolet radiation*. While certain types of tumors in dogs can be caused by prolonged exposure of lightly pigmented skin to ultraviolet radiation, it is far less common than in humans. In fact, the vast majority of skin neoplasms in dogs appears to arise spontaneously, possibly due to an undetermined causative agent. *Breeding* is another variable that may relate to the numbers and types of skin tumors seen in certain dogs. Cutaneous neoplasms appear to be twice as common in purebred dogs compared to mixed breeds. Additionally, certain breeds, such as boxers, and related breeds such as Boston terriers and bull terriers, are predisposed to develop *mastocytoma*, a specific type of skin neoplasm.

A final variable in development of cutaneous tumors in dogs is *age*. With the exception of a few types of tumors, the incidence of tumors increases proportionally with the age of the animal. Although the precise reason for this is not fully understood, many experts believe it is related to the aging of the immune system. The normal defense mechanisms that the body uses to destroy abnormal or neoplastic cells are weakened with age, as are many other systems in the body. Others believe it is as a result of an accumulation of carcinogen exposure, such as sunlight or pesticides.

Cutaneous neoplasms generally fall into one of two categories: those arising from the skin itself, and those arising in the underlying soft tissue. Both are common in the dog and are covered in this chapter.

## Tumors of the Skin

### Basal Cell Tumors

Basal cell tumors account for between 5 to 10 percent of skin tumors in the dog. They arise from a primitive population of cells in the skin that eventually matures into hair follicles or sweat glands. The average age of dogs with basal cell tumors is approximately seven years; cocker spaniels and poodles have a predilection to develop these neoplasms. These tumors are generally small (less than 2 cm), usually single, and are not attached to underlying structures. They are most commonly seen on the head and neck, are solid, and, occasionally, have an ulcerated surface. Under the pathologists' microscope, basal cell tumors have many different appearances and are often classified by the pattern in which the neoplastic cells are arranged. However, all types of basal cell tumors are invariably benign in the dog. If excision or removal is complete, these tumors will not regrow, and the prognosis is good.

### Hair Follicle Tumors

Neoplasms that arise from cells that make up the hair follicles are fairly common in dogs, but rare in other domestic animals. These neoplasms are solitary, dome-shaped nodules that arise beneath the epidermis, may have an ulcerated surface and are usually freely movable underneath the skin. Some types of hair follicle tumors may contain a central pore, which, when squeezed, exudes a yellowish-white, greasy material. There are numerous types of hair follicle tumors that are classified by the major type of neoplastic cells seen, and the degree to which they resemble normal hair follicles. *Trichoepitheliomas*, for example, are composed of well-defined follicle-like structures which, in some areas, may even grow hair. This neoplasm contains cells from all layers of the follicle. *Pilomatrixomas* are more primitive neoplasms arising primarily only from those cells which generate the hair shaft itself. There are many other types of follicular tumors in dogs which arise from other specialized parts of the hair follicles.

While the cellular origin of these neoplasms is important to the veterinary pathologist as a way to categorize them, it is generally of little importance to the animal and its owner, as the vast majority of follicular tumors are benign in nature. In a small number of cases these tumors may be malignant, infiltrating and destroying adjacent tissue until they are removed by a surgeon. Metastasis to visceral organs is exceedingly rare.

### Sebaceous Gland Tumors

*Sebaceous glands* are found in association with hair follicles in the dog. Their secretory product, *sebum,* has numerous responsibilities in the skin, including minimizing water loss, decreasing entry of microorganisms, and keeping the skin soft and pliable. Sebaceous gland tumors are considered the most common epithelial tumor in the dog. The average age of dogs and cats developing these neoplasms is 9 to 10 years. Cocker spaniels and poodles appear to be predisposed. They arise as single or multiple, cauliflower-like growths on the animal up to a centimeter in diameter, with malignant tumors ranging in size as high as ten centimeters. They can arise anywhere on the body, including the eyelids, which have a large population of modified sebaceous glands. The thorax is also a common site in the dog. As is the case with follicular tumors, squeezing these masses may result in production of a yellowish, greasy fluid, which is composed of accumulated sebum and dead tumor cells.

There are two distinct types of benign sebaceous gland proliferations in the dog, *hyperplasia* and *adenoma*. In *sebaceous hyperplasia,* there is a rapid proliferation of these glands leading to a nodular mass. The glands are well-formed and properly oriented around the ducts which carry their secretions into the hair follicle, and are not considered neoplastic by nature. *Adenomas,* which are neoplasms, are characterized by loss of normal architecture, i.e. the glands are well-formed, but are not oriented around ducts; their secretions have nowhere to go. Adenomas may be accompanied by inflammation resulting from extrusion of sebum into the surrounding dermis. Complete surgical excision of either of these lesions results in a cure, although similar tumors may appear at a later time in other areas of the dog's body.

*Sebaceous adenocarcinomas* are less common and have a higher rate of internal, or visceral metastasis. These tumors can metastasize to local lymph nodes, or to the lung, with potentially fatal results. In the case of these and all other malignant tumors, life-threatening complications can often be prevented by observant owners who have skin tumors on their pets removed in a timely fashion and examined.

### Apocrine Sweat Gland Tumors

Apocrine sweat glands, a second type of sweat gland in the dog, uncommonly become neoplastic. Apocrine glands are similar to sweat glands in human skin; however, in dogs they are minimally functional. These tumors generally occur in dogs over eight years of age, regardless of sex. Golden retrievers and cocker spaniels have been reported to be predisposed to these neoplasms. The tumors are generally single and can appear anywhere on the body. In opposition to most types of skin tumors in the dog, malignant apocrine gland tumors (*adenocarcinomas*) appear to be more common than their benign counterparts. Although visceral metastasis is rare, aggressive malignancies can extend deep into underlying subcutaneous tissues and muscle, often requiring extensive surgery. A common non-neoplastic involving apocrine glands is an apocrine *cyst*. Apocrine glands often become swollen and distended, elevating the overlying skin and feeling like a small nodule. This will happen whenever the duct connecting the gland to the skin surface becomes plugged. Removal of these cysts is a simple procedure and completely curative.

## Tumors of Modified Glands of the Perianal Area

In certain areas of the dog's body, there are certain types of sebaceous and apocrine glands which have been modified both in form and function. The mammary gland is an apocrine gland which has been modified to produce a copious amount of a highly specialized secretion — milk. In addition, these glands rapidly enlarge and become functional only when pregnancy hormones are in abundance. It is outside the scope of this chapter to discuss the many variants of mammary neoplasms that arise in the dog. Suffice it to say that mammary neoplasms are extremely common.

The perianal area contains several types of modified glands such as the *circumanal* or *perianal* glands which are modified sebaceous glands. They are found in largest numbers around the anus, but may also extend along the abdomen and flanks of the dog, and rarely along the back. Circumanal glands arise from cells of the hair follicles in the developing fetus, but their shape and function changes as the puppy develops. These glands are best developed in male dogs, where *androgens*, or male hormones, appear to stimulate their development. These glands are present in females, but are less well-developed, as *estrogen* appears to inhibit them. Circumanal glands appear to be involved in sex scent recognition.

Tumors of the circumanal glands are extremely common in the dog, especially in uncastrated males. They are reported to be the third most common tumor in dogs overall (behind mast cell tumors, which we will discuss later, and mammary tumors.) They usually appear as a nodule lateral to the anus, which, in severe cases, may totally encircle the anus, giving a "napkin-ring" appearance. They often are large and ulcerate, and may cause straining and difficulty in defecation. The vast majority of these tumors are benign. Complete surgical excision is usually curative; castration of intact males will decrease the possibility of development of tumors in adjacent glands. One possible surgical complication is the inadvertent cutting of the nerves which control the muscle of the anal sphincter. Should this occur, an incontinent dog may be the end result. This is why it is important to remove these tumors at an early date while they are still small.

Malignant circumanal gland tumors have been reported to comprise 1 to 20 percent of all neoplasms of circumanal glands; however, the true incidence is probably at the low end of this figure. They appear to be more common in females than in males. They can metastasize to internal lymph nodes and organs surrounding the pelvic canal and may be life-threatening if not detected early. A second type of canine neoplasm arises from modified apocrine glands of the anal sacs. *Anal sacs*, or *anal glands* as they are often referred to, are paired structures on either side of the anus which contain a foul-smelling fluid. When excited or frightened, some animals may inadvertently squeeze these sacs, resulting in a quite unpleasant, fetid odor. (Skunk anal sacs are the best-developed in the animal kingdom.) The proposed function of the fluid produced by these structures is to lubricate the anus during the passage of feces.

These glands often develop malignant tumors in aged (over 10 years) female dogs. They present a diagnostic challenge due to their propensity to grow *forward* into the pelvic canal, rather than outward underneath the skin of the anus. Hence, a dog with only a small perianal nodule may have extensive secondary tumors throughout the abdomen. These neoplasms cause problems other than abdominal metastasis; they can also secrete hormones which upset the calcium regulation of the body, markedly raising the blood levels of calcium (hypercalcemia). Hypercalcemia may lead to additional clinical signs in these animals such as decreased appetite, excessive thirst and urination, and weakness. While complete removal of the tumor may be curative, often the surgery is performed too late, and only after extensive metastasis has occurred. There is a poor prognosis in animals with this neoplasm.

### Ceruminous Gland Tumors

Modified apocrine glands that line the ear canal are *ceruminous glands*. These glands produce *cerumen*, the characteristic dark brown material often referred to as *wax* which is composed of glandular secretions and epidermal debris. Ceruminous gland tumors are small, cauliflower-like growths which are often connected to the skin of the ear canal by a variably thick stalk. They are commonly associated with ear infections leading some authors to suggest that they may arise in areas of chronic inflammation. Benign ceruminous gland tumors are more common than malignant tumors; surgical excision is often curative — as long as the surgeon is careful to remove the factors which predispose their growth, such as chronic infection.

### Tumors of the Epidermis

We will discuss two main groups of neoplasms which arise in the composing the outside layer of the skin, or the *epidermis* — **papillomas** and **squamous cell carcinomas**. *Papillomas*, often referred to as "warts," are commonly seen in dogs and other animals (as well as in humans), and may arise either as a result of viral infection, or spontaneously. In young dogs, *papillomaviruses* may infect the skin, resulting in the growth of single to multiple white, firm, cauliflower-like growths, particularly around the face and neck; they are especially common in the mouth and gums, although they may be found anywhere on the body. While large numbers of these tumors may be unsightly or even cause difficulty in eating, they most often regress with time. Papillomas arising in older dogs, however, may arise spontaneously or rarely, due to other less common forms of papillomaviruses. Tumors arising in older dogs rarely regress and require surgical excision. These tumors are invariably benign and carry a good prognosis; however, they occasionally act as sites for development of malignant tumors of other types.

*Squamous cell carcinomas* may be found in all areas of the skin, but are most common in the poorly pigmented, sparsely-haired areas of the body - ears, lips, trunk and scrotum. The reason that most tumors arise in this area is that the most important carcinogenic stimulus for their development is ultraviolet radiation. These tumors develop slowly, progressing from a small, "precancerous" lesion to one which is confined to the epidermis, and finally resulting in a malignant neoplasm which infiltrates deeply into subjacent dermis, fat, and muscle, and may metastasize to local lymph nodes and the lung.

The visual appearance of these tumors depends on their *chronicity*, or the length of time that they have been present. These tumors, when detected, often appear as scabby, ulcerated, reddish plaque-like masses, and may be mistaken for areas which the dog has been scratching. When unresponsive to therapy, a surgical biopsy reveals its true identity. White, poorly-haired areas of the body which are exposed to sunlight — such as the tips of white ears, the face, and occasionally the abdomen or scrotum of dogs which spend a significant portion of time on concrete runs — are most commonly affected.

Although this is a malignant neoplasm, early and complete surgical excision is often curative. Larger, more chronic lesions may have already spread to nearby lymph nodes or internal organs by the time surgery is performed, and may result in the death of the animal.

### Melanomas

*Melanomas* are common neoplasms in man but less so in the dog and cat. They are derived from *melanocytes*, or the cells which manufacture pigment in the skin. Normally, melanocytes are most numerous in heavily pigmented areas of the skin, however, neoplasms of melanocytes may arise anywhere on the body. These tumors arise in older animals, and appear to be more common in males. They are most common in heavily pigmented breeds of dogs, such as Scottish terriers, Boston terriers, Dobermans, schnauzers and poodles. Melanomas are extremely varied in their appearance, and can range from small polyp-like gray, brown, or black fleshy tumors, to large darkened, ulcerated plaques, or just about anything in between. They may be single or multiple in origin.

Benign cutaneous melanomas (*melanocytomas*) are commonly seen in older dogs over the age of eight years anywhere on the body. They are similar to *nevi* or "moles," which are common blemishes of human skin. They may affect the epidermis, the dermis, or both; however, excision of these tumors is generally curative. Although benign melanomas in humans occasionally change into a malignant form, this transformation is not well documented in domestic animals.

*Malignant melanomas*, although less common than their benign counterparts, commonly result in the death of the animal due to a combination of infiltration of adjacent tissue and metastasis to internal organs. Melanomas arising in certain sites — such as the digits, oral cavity and lips, and scrotum. — are often malignant. Ulceration is a common finding in these tumors.

Due to the inherent difficulties in assessing the benign or malignant potential of melanomas by visual inspection in the dog, it is highly recommended that all darkly pigmented neoplasms of the dog skin be removed and biopsied.

### Cutaneous Histiocytomas

*Histiocytomas* are among the most common skin tumors in the dog, but are seen in no other animal species. Histiocytomas, as their name implies, are neoplasms made up of *histiocytes*, a type of white blood cell living in the tissues rather than the blood. The cause of this tumor is unknown, although some pathologists consider it to be more of a local inflammatory lesion (in which spontaneous regression would be likely) than a distinct neoplastic entity. They are rapidly growing neoplasms, arising within 1-4 weeks, dome-shaped and often red and ulcerated, explaining why they get the name "strawberry tumor." They generally appear as a solitary tumor on the head, especially the ear, but also may occur on the legs, neck, and abdomen. Although any dog can develop them. they are most commonly seen in purebred dogs such as boxers, cocker spaniels, dachshunds, and great Danes

Histiocytomas are most commonly seen in young dogs less than two years of age in which case spontaneous regression is often seen. Regression is far less common in dogs four years and older. There is no malignant variant of this tumor.

### Mastocytoma

In some reviews, *mast cell tumors* are the single most common skin tur̄ the dog, comprising from between 7-20 percent of all skin tumors. Mast cells, primarily located around vessels, are a normal component of skin which manufacture substances such as histamine and heparin, and are involved in allergic reactions. They are largely responsible for the swelling and itching associated with allergic reactions such as hives. These neoplasms are most common in dogs eight to 10 years of age, with Boston terriers, bull terriers, and Labrador retrievers being predisposed. Most mast cell tumors appear as small dome-shaped red "buttons" which may arise anywhere on the dog's body, and may grow up to several centimeters in diameter appearing as a large, thickened, ulcerated plaque on the abdomen or flanks.

Mast cell tumors can behave in various ways in the dog. Some are benign in nature; complete excision of these tumors is curative. However, a significant proportion of mast cell tumors will invade deep tissues and may even metastasize to other organs, ultimately resulting in the death of the animal. Additionally, mast cell tumors have been associated with peptic ulcers in the dog, due to the manufacture and release of abnormally large amounts of histamine by the neoplastic cells. Increased levels of histamine cause elevated acid secretion in the stomachs of these animals.

### Plasmacytoma

*Plasmacytomas* are cutaneous tumors of dog skin, that recently seem to be increasingly diagnosed the dog. *Plasma cells* are responsible for production of antibodies throughout the body. Neoplasms of plasma cells also resemble mast cell tumors or histiocytomas (small, red, dome-shaped nodules), and are most commonly seen on the digits, lips and ears. The average age of affected dogs is 10 years, and cocker spaniels appear to have a predilection for developing these tumors. The vast majority of these neoplasms are benign, and complete excision carries a good prognosis.

## Tumors of the Soft Tissues

These tumors often involve the skin, but by a strict definition, they usually arise from the subcutaneous tissues.

### Lipoma

*Lipomas* are neoplasms arising from proliferation of adipocytes, or fat cells. Most lipomas are considered neoplasms due to their appearance as a lump underneath the skin; however a small percentage invade adjacent tissues, and malignant tumors of fat, known as liposarcomas are rarely seen. Lipomas are the most common soft tissue tumor in the dog, accounting for 8 to 10 percent of all reported skin tumors. cocker spaniels, dachshunds, Labrador retrievers, and weimeraners report the highest incidence of these tumors. They are most common in older dogs, and often appear over the thorax, sternum, forelimbs, and the abdomen.

Lipomas appear as flabby, fleshy nodules beneath the skin, which are generally soft and freely movable. They may range up to 30 centimeters in diameter. Surgical excision is curative in the vast majority of lipomas although if a significant proportion of these neoplasms remain, regrowth may occur. *Infiltrative lipomas*, benign tumors which infiltrate into adjacent tissues (primarily muscles), pose a special problem. As complete excision is rarely accomplished, these tumors may result in significant loss of function in affected animals due to mechanical disturbance and/or pain. *Liposarcomas* are uncommon malignancies in the dog. They are primarily infiltrative in nature, and may result in destruction of adjacent tissue. Metastasis is rare.

### Fibroma

*Fibromas* are neoplasms of fibrous connective tissue that often arise in the dermis or subcutaneous tissue of older dogs. This type of neoplasm does not appear to have any sex or breed predilection. Fibromas appear as hard, discrete lumps or dome-shaped masses in the skin of dogs which are easily removed and have a good prognosis.

### Fibrosarcomas

These malignant tumors also arise in the skin of dogs, most commonly in the trunk and extremities. They appear as irregularly-shaped nodular, poorly demarcated neoplasms which blend with adjacent tissues and may be ulcerated. These tumors grow rapidly and aggressively into adjacent tissues, and metastasize in approximately 25 percent of cases, largely to the lungs. Due to their infiltrative nature, surgical excision is rarely complete, and regrowth of these tumors is common. Prognoses for these tumors range from guarded to poor.

### Tumors of Blood Vessels

Another common benign tumor of the skin and subcutaneous tissue is the *hemangioma*, which arises from blood vessels in the skin or any other organ. There is no breed or sex predilection in the dog, and the average age of affected animals is nine years. They are commonly seen in the dermis of the face, leg, and flanks, and are usually single. Hemangiomas appear as dark, raised, fleshy nodules in the skin and bleed profusely if traumatized. They are generally easy to remove, and when completely excised, do not recur.

As with other soft tissue tumors, there is a malignant variant (*hemangiosarcoma*) which is one of the most common malignancies in the dog. *Primary hemangiosarcomas* (which originate in the skin) are very rare. Most hemangiosarcomas in the skin represent metastasis from a tumor which has grown in an internal organ (usually in the spleen). German shepherds are the breed most often affected, with males more commonly affected. They have a high rate of metastasis, and generally offer a poor prognosis.

### Cutaneous Spindle Cell Sarcomas

This term is used to describe a group of three types of soft tissue neoplasms which are low-grade malignant tumors that infiltrate extensively, but rarely metastasize. The group includes *neurofibrosarcomas* and *Schwannomas* (tumors of the cells comprising nerves), and *hemangiopericytoma* (a tumor arising from proliferation of pericytes, cells which surround blood vessels). The reason that these three tumors are grouped together is that they are almost indistinguishable to the pathologist underneath the microscope in their appearance and they all behave in a similar fashion. Only by using an *electron microscope*, which looks at the details of a single cell, can the three tumors be positively identified.

These tumors primarily occur in the extremities of older dogs, and have been reported to represent from 3.2-4.2 percent of cutaneous neoplasms in the dog. The average age of affected dogs is 10 years, and females appear to be more commonly affected. These are generally slow-growing tumors, but they may grow to 20 centimeters in size or larger. They appear as a large, firm mass which is often hairless and ulcerated. These tumors have a high rate of recurrence after surgery due to their infiltrative nature, although metastasis is exceedingly rare.

# Glossary of Terms

**A**

**Abrasion-** Removal of superficial epidermis resulting in weeping and crusting.

**Abscess-**Localized accumulation of pus.

**Acanthosis nigricans-**Describes increased pigment and thickening of skin often found in armpits.

**Acariasis-**An infestation caused by a mite.

**Acemannan-**A potent stimulator of the immune system derived from aloe.

**Acne-**Describes comedone or blackhead in skin.

**Actinic-**Caused by sunlight.

**Adenoma-**Benign tumor of a gland.

**Adnexa-**The epithelial structures of the skin which arise from the epidermis: the hair follicle and the sebaceous, apocrine and eccrine glands.

**Allergen-**Substance capable of inducing an allergic reaction.

**Allergy-**An excessive immune response to a common substance.

**Alopecia-**The loss of hair.

**Anagen-**Growth stage of hair cycle.

**Anaphylactoid-**Anaphylaxis like, does not involve antibodies.

**Anaphylaxis-**Severe hypersensitive (allergic) reactions involving multiple systems (primarily in man and cats-respiratory,dogs-liver) involving the immune system and antibodies.

**Anibodies-**A group of proteins produced by b lymphocytes that have the ability to bind antigens; they are a component of the humoral immune system.

**Antibody-**A type of serum protein known as a globulin produced by lymphocytes in response to an antigen (example, antibody is the protective substance produced by the body after vaccination--the vaccine is the antigen).

**Antigen-**A high molecular weight protein or protein-polysaccharide which when foreign to the animal stimulates the formation of specific antibody (example, a vaccine serves as the antigen to simulate the production of protective antibodies).

**Anti-Nuclear Antibody test (ANA)-**A diagnostic test that detects the presence of auto-antibodies against inside components of the body's cells.

**Apocrine gland-**A gland attached to the upper portion of the hair follicle by a long duct; in normal dogs and cats produce a viscid secretion which is responsible for body odors and may be important for the integrity of the horny cell layer.

**Atopy-**Sometimes referred to as allergic inhalant dermatitis or hay fever, occurs in animals that are hereditarily predisposed to develop antibodies (Immunoglobulin E, IgE) to normal environmental proteins causing a hypersensitivity reaction.

**Atrophy-**Wasting away or decrease in size of cell, tissue, organ or part.

**Auto-immunity-**The direction of an immune response against normal components of the body.

**Auto-reactive-**Cells or molecules that are programmed to attack the body.

**Axillary-**Armpit region.

## B

**Basal cell layer-**The cell layer of the epidermis adjacent to the dermis. The keratinocytes in the basal cell layer are the only cells which normally are able to divide and produce new keratinocytes.

**Basement membrane-**The region where the epidermis is attached to the dermis.

**Benign-**Mild or not serious as it pertains to diseases or tumors.

**Bioflavonoid-**A compound derived from plant polyphenols with myriad anti-inflammatory properties. Examples include quercitin and catechin.

**Biopsy samples-**Small pieces of tissue that are removed for microscopic examination.

**Bromelain-**An enzyme isolated from pineapple that helps combat inflammation in the body.

**Bullous Pemphigoid-**An auto-immune blistering disease that produces lesions at mucocutaneous junctions.

## C

**Catagen-**The stage between the end of anagen and the beginning of telogen.

**Cerumen-**Waxlike combined excretions of apocrine, sebaceous and epithelial cells.

**Co-enzyme Q-**A nutritional supplement related to vitamin $K_1$ that works as an antioxidant and immune stimulant in the body.

**Collagen-**A fibrous protein which is the major component of the dermis.

**Collie Nose-**A pseudonym for discoid lupus erythematosus.

**Comedone-**Blackhead, plugged hair follicle or duct, acne.

**Corticosteroid-**A steroid produced by the adrenal cortex, either synthetic, exogenous (prednisone) or made by the body, endogenous (cortisol), AKA glucocorticoids.

**Crust-**An accumulation of dried pus, blood, or scale adhered to the skin and hair, AKA scab.

**Cryosurgery-**Therapy by freezing affected tissue, using liquid nitrogen. Damage cancerous cells by repeating freeze-thaw cycles. For small localized lesions.

**Cutaneous Asthenia/Ehlers-Danlos syndrome-**A group of congenital, hereditary disorders involving weakness and hyperextensibility of the skin.

**Cutaneous Lupus Erythematosus-**An auto-immune disease that is a cross-over between systemic lupus erythematosus and discoid lupus erythematosus.

**Cutis-**The epidermis and the dermis.

**Cytosis-**Increase in number, usually with a cell prefix, leukocytosis.

## D

**Dalmatian bronzing syndrome-**Disorder seen in Dalmatians in which the have a brown discoloration along the back.

**Demodicosis-**Infestation with the mite, Demodex.

**Dermatitis-**Inflammation of the skin.

**Dermatomyositis-**Inflammatory condition of skin, muscle and sometimes blood vessels usually developing in collies and Shetland sheep dogs.

**Dermatophyte-**A keratin-loving fungus which grows in the hair follicles and, especially in cats, in the horny cell layer; disease caused by dermatophytes is known as either dermatophytosis or "ringworm".

**Dermis-**The layer of skin immediately beneath the epidermis that provides it with nutrients and support which is composed of collagen, elastin and glycosaminoglycans.

247

**Dermoid sinus**-Most commonly seen in Rhodesian ridgebacks, an abnormal congenital tract connecting the skin surface with the down as deep as the spinal cord.

**Desmosome**-The site at which keratinocytes are connected.

**Diabetic dermatopathy**-A rare metabolic skin disorder often associated with increased glucagon levels and, occasionally, a glucagon-secreting tumor.

**Dimethylglycine**-An amino acid that seems to enhance the function of the immune system and the cardiovascular system; not currently considered "essential" in dogs or cats.

**Dipsea**-Thirst or water intake. **-Polydipsea**= increased thirst or water intake.

**Dirofilariasis**-Heartworm infection. When microfilariae are found in the dermis, the condition is referred to as cutaneous dirofilariasis.

**Discoid Lupus Erythematosus**-A benign, facially-oriented auto-immune disease.

**Dorsum**-The back, top of pelvis, in the case of pets, the top.

**Drug eruption**-An immune-mediated reaction to a medication.

**E**

**Eccrine gland**-A gland present in the foot pads in dogs and cats whose secretion is watery and it is believed to assist in increasing traction.

**Echinacea**-A plant that provides several ingredients known to fight inflammation and infections in the body. It is considered an herbal remedy.

**Eicosapentaenoic acid (EPA)**-A polyunsaturated fatty acid found in fish oils, together with docosahexaenoic acid (DHA). Can be made in the body from alpha-linolenic acid if proper enzymes are present.

**Elastin**-A protein that allows the dermis to stretch and retract.

**Electromyogram**-The record of the changes in electrical potential of muscle obtained by surface or needle electrodes inserted into muscle or by stimulation of the nerve.

**Emollient**-Softening agent.

**Endocrine**-Refers to a system composed of organs that secrete a substance, known as hormones, that has a specific effect on another organ; secreting within, or dispersing into circulation; subjected to complex multi-feedback regulation.

**Eosinophilic granuloma**-A disorder of dogs (i.e., huskies) believed to be immune-mediated, with collagen breakdown and tissue eosinophilia.

**Eosinophilic granuloma complex**-A group of three separate inflammatory conditions (indolent ulcer, eosinophilic plaque, and linear [collagenolytic] granuloma) in cats.

**Epidermal collarette**-A circular rim of scale.

**Epidermal cyst**-A cyst derived from the epidermis.

**Epidermis**-The outer layer of the skin which is composed primarily of keratinocytes; arranged in distinct layers; the major protective barrier of the skin.

**Erythema**- Redness of the skin, seen in inflammation.

**Erythema multiforme**-A severe skin disorder which is a presumably immune-mediated reaction to a drug, microbe, or other unknown agent.

**Essential Fatty Acids**-Fatty Acids that must be supplied in the diet or deficiencies will result including cis-linoleic acid in the dog and cis-linoleic and arachidonic acid in the cat.

**Etiology**-The cause of the disease.

**Excoriation**-Removal of the superficial layer of the skin by biting or scratching.

## F

**Folliculitis**-An inflammatory reaction directed against hair follicles.

**Furunculosis**-A deep skin infection in which a ruptured hair follicle results in an inflammatory reaction.

## G

**Gamma-linolenic acid (GLA)**-A polyunsaturated fatty acid found in borage oil, evening primrose oil and black currant seed oil; it can be made in the body from cis-linoleic acid if proper enzymes are present.

**Generic dog food disease**-Named after a nutritionally related skin problem associated with the feeding of generic dog foods; presumably due to a zinc imbalance caused by the high cereal (fiber, phytates) content.

**Genetic**-Inherited.

**Glucocorticoids**-A group of hormonal drugs with multiple functions including to induce immunosuppression, suppress inflammation , treat shock with many adverse effects.

**Glycosaminoglycans**-A complex molecule that attracts water and maintains the normal homeostasis of the dermis.

**Granuloma**-A well-circumscribed tissue reaction composed mainly of cells from the macrophage system.

**Gynecomastia**-Enlarged breasts, nipples and/or clitoris.

## H

**Hair**-One of the fine, long appendages of the skin, composed of keratin.

**Hair follicle**-The adnexal structure that produces hair shafts.

**Hepatocutaneous syndrome**-A netabolic skin disease associated by liver disease. AKA necrolytic migratory erythema.

**Hepatoid gland adenoma (perianal adenoma)**-A benign tumor of modified sebaceous glands commonly found around the anus of dogs .

**Histiocyte**-*see* macrophage.

**Histiocytoma**-AKA strawberry tumor, a common tumor of young dogs that looks aggressive but is almost always benign.

**Histopathology**-A microscopic exam of diseased tissue.

**Homeopathy**-A form of therapy using exceptionally small doses of extracts to treat disease that, in full doses, would cause similar symptoms.

**Horny cell layer**-The most superficial layer of the epidermis, cells in this layer are long, thin and devoid of a nucleus; provides the structural barrier of the skin.

**Hot Spots**-Localized areas of self-induced trauma that are secondarily infected, usually moist, weepy and hot due to inflammation, irritation and itching.

**Humectant**-Moisturizing agent..

**Hyperadrenocorticism**-*see* Cushing's disease.

**Hyperkeratosis**-An increased thickness of the horny layer of the skin often of the footpads.

**Hyperpigmentation**-Darkening of the skin caused by an increase in melanin pigment in skin.

**Hypersensitivity**-An excessive immune response to a substance. The four classic hypersensitivity reactions are immediate (**Type I**; e.g., allergic inhalant dermatitis); cytotoxic (**Type II**; e.g., pemphigus); immune complexes (**Type III**; lupus erythematosus), and delayed, cell mediated (**Type IV** contact allergy).

**Hyperthermia**-High temperature; therapy by administering local current field radio frequency at 50° C, for 30-60 seconds; works in only small lesions.

**Hypothyroidism**-An endocrine disorder characterized by a decrease in the amount of circulating thyroid horlmones.

## I-J

**Ichthyosis**-A group of hereditary, often congenital, skin diseases, in which the epidermis is covered with scales.

**Immune complexes**-A bound unit of an antibody and antigen that may circulate and deposit in tissue resulting in inflammation.

**Immune system**-A complex organization of cells and molecules designed to protect the body.

**Immunodeficiency**-The lack of an effective immune response.

**Immunofluorescent**-A complex diagnostic tool that accentuates the particular immune molecule being studied.

**Immunosuppression**-The inhibition of the body's immune system.

**Impetigo**-A superficial bacterial infection often seen on the underside of puppies.

**Infiltrate**-Penetrate, usually describing a diseased state in tissue

**Inflammation**-A tissue reaction to injury involving pain, heat, redness, swelling and occasional loss of function.

**Inguinal**-Groin region (the area between the thighs).

**Itch**-*see* Pruritus.

**Juvenile cellulitis**-A condition in which the face and head of young pups becomes inflamed and swollen that remarkably responds to short-term immunosuppressive therapy.

## K

**Keratinization disorder**-A disorder involving increased layers of scale on the skin surface, AKA seborrhea.

**Keratinous**-Tough fibrous proteins that are present in all epidermal and adnexal structures; make up the majority of volume of the horny cell layer and hair shaft.

**Keratinocytes**-The cells of the epidermis that are held together by desmosomes.

## L

**Langerhans cell**-A cell with long arms, interspersed between keratinocytes. that play a major role in the immunologic barrier of the skin.

**Lanugo**-Fine, down or woolly hair.

**Lentigo**-A freckle or lentil shaped pigmented spot.

**Lesion**--An overused term describing any diseased or abnormal tissue

**Lethal acrodermatitis**-An inherited disorder with some similarities to zinc deficiency.

**Leukocyte**-White blood cell; consists of neutrophil, lymphocyte, monocyte, eosinophil and basophil.

**Lichenification**-Thickening and hardening of the skin usually from friction or chronic trauma.

**Lichenoid**-Grossly refers to a flat-topped skin lesion and, microscopically, a dense band at the dermoepidermal junction.

**Lupus erythematosus**-An auto-immune disease; involving skin only, discoid or, if it involves at least one other organ system with supportive lab results, it is systemic.

**Lymphocytes**-One type of white blood cell that is part of the immune system.

# M

**Macrophage**-Large cells that are phagocytic, in skin, AKA histiocyte.

**Macule**-A discreet flat spot where the skin has changed color from pigment changes, bleeding, or inflammation.

**Malassezia dermatitis**-A greasy, skin infection caused by the yeast, *Malassezia pachydermatis* (previously known as *Pityrosporon canis*).

**Mange**-A clinical disorder caused by mites.

**Mast cell tumor**-A potentially malignant tumor of mast cells, which are the cells believed to be the cause of Type I hypersensitivity (Atopy, hay-fever).

**Melanocyte**-A cell in the basal cell layer of the epidermis that produces a red or black pigment (melanin) which is packaged in granules and taken up by adjacent keratinocytes; responsible for hair and skin color. In contrast to humans, melanin in dogs and cats plays only a secondary role in photoprotection.

**Melanoma**-A melanocyte tumor.

**Miliary dermatitis**-A papular, scaly skin disorder most often seen in cats usually caused by allergy.

**Monounsaturated fatty acids**-Fatty acids that have one double bond, such as oleic acid found in olive and canola oils.

**Mucinosis**-A rare skin condition caused by the accumulation of mucin, a stringy, sticky substance found in the dermis most commonly reported in Chinese shar- peis and Doberman pinschers.

**Mucocutaneous junctions**-The zones of the body where the skin meets the lining of the body's orifices(i.e., lips, eyelids, anus).

**Mycetoma**-An infection characterized by swelling, draining sinuses, and granules involving the skin, subcutaneous tissue, fascia, and bone.

**Mycosis**-Any disease caused by a fungus.

**Mycosis fungoides**-A lymphoma involving a subset of lymphocytes (T-cells) characterized by a red scaly rash that evolves into cutaneous tumors. Named because the clinical appearance of these tumors in humans was said to resemble mushrooms.

**Myiasis**-Invasion of tissues by flies or their larva (maggots).

**Myositis**-Inflammation of muscles.

# N

**Nasal Solar Dermatitis**-A pseudonym for discoid lupus erythematosus.

**Necrolytic migratory erythema**-*see* Hepatocutaneous syndrome.

**Neurodermatitis (psychogenic alopecia)**-A condition caused by obsessive and somewhat compulsive licking

**Nevus (cutaneous hamartoma)**-A general term describing any congenital lesion or discolored patch of skin which is categorized by tissue of origin (e.g., epidermal, vascular, melanocytic, organoid).

**Niacinamide**-A derivative of niacin that has been used in the treatment of some immune-mediated skin disorders.

**Nodule**-A discreet, firm, solid elevation in the skin larger than 1 cm extending deeper into the skin.

**Non-self**-Molecules and cells that do not belong to a specific individual.

# O

**Otitis**-Inflammation of the ear, classified by location; **-externa**-external ear canal; **-interna**-inner ear; **-media**-middle ear.

**Otodectic mange**-Infestation with *Otodectes cynotis*, the common ear mite.

## P

**Panniculitis**-An inflammatory reaction in the subcutaneous fat.

**Panniculus**-The layer of fat located between the dermis and underlying muscle, the tissue directly below the skin.

**Pansteatitis**-An inflammatory disorder of the fat in cats, caused by a relative deficiency of vitamin E.

**Papilloma**-A common skin tumor AKA wart. that is not induced by viruses like those that cause papillomatosis.

**Papule**-A small, firm elevation in the skin, often pink or red, caused by inflammation.

**Pathology**-The study of disease, histo-= microscopic study of disease.

**Pemphigus complex**-The group of four pemphigus diseases that share a similar disease mechanism; derived from the Greek word for "blister". -**Erythematosus**-a benign form of pemphigus foliaceus., or a cross-over disease between foliaceus and lupus erythematosus. -**Foliaceus**-The most common form that produces superficial vesicles and crusts. -**Vegetans**-the rarest form with lesions similar, but less severe, than vulgaris. -**Vulgaris**-The most severe and deep form that produces deep ulcers on the body, mouth and mucous membranes.

**Penia**-Suffix meaning decrease in cell number, i.e.,lymphopenia.

**Phagia**-Suffix meaning appetite, polyphagia, increased appetite.

**Phagocytosis**-Cell ingestion.

**Philia**-Suffix meaning increase cell number, neutrophilia.

**Photochemotherapy**-Intravenous injection of photosensitive drug, which binds to cancerous cells, followed by selective wave length of light. Theoretically, it will kill cancer cells selectively, but the result is variable. Since it can be used in relatively small areas, pretreatment to reduce the size of the lesion may be necessary. Availability is limited.

**Photosensitivity**-Abnormal skin reaction to ultraviolet light, mainly UVB, which involves immune responses.

**Pigment**-The dark, or color-producing molecules of the skin.

**Pinocytosis**-Cell drinking.

**Pododermatitis**-An inflammatory condition of the feet and toes.

**Poliosis**-The premature graying of hair.

**Poly**-Prefix indicating multiple or increased amount, i.e., polydipsea.

**Polyunsaturated Fatty Acids (PUFA)**-Fatty acids with two or more double bonds present in the molecule. An example is linoleic acid found in vegetable oils.

**Prognosis**-Predictability for the outcome of the disease.

**Pruritus**-The medical term for itch, an unpleasant cutaneous sensation provoking the desire to scratch, rub, lick or chew.

**Psychogenic alopecia**-*see* neurodermatitis.

**Pustule**-A small, discreet elevation in the skin filled with pus.

**Pyoderma**-Literally, pus in the skin, this is an extremely common skin condition characterized by the influx of neutrophils(pus cells). Generally, used to describe any form of skin infection.

## R

**Retinoids**-A group of synthetic Vitamin A derivatives, notably isotretinoin (Accutane) and etretinate (Tegison).

**Rhabditic dermatitis**-A term for the condition caused by infestation of the nematode *Pelodera (Rhabditis) strongyloides*.

**Ringworm**-*see* dermatophytosis.

# S

**Scabies**-A severely itchy disorder caused by the mite, *Sarcoptic scabieii*.

**Scales**-Large, loose flakes of the horny cell layer. In humans, the presence of scales in haired skin is called dandruff.

**Scar**-An area of fibrous tissue that has replaced damaged skin and subcutaneous tissue.

**Schnauzer comedo syndrome**-A skin disorder usually seen down the back, believed to be a keratinization disorder in which keratin plugs develop in hair follicles, that may be aggravated by frequent clipping.

**Sebaceous adenitis**-A congenito-hereditary, presumably immune-mediated disorder tin which the sebaceous glands are selectively attacked. leaving patches of hairless and scaly skin.

**Sebaceous gland**-A gland attached to the hair follicle that is connected to the hair follicle by a short duct; produces sebum, a secretion composed primarily of fatty material and, to lesser extent, protein.

**Sebaceous glands**-Prominent in the haired skin of pets glands that secrete sebum and are attached to the hair follicle by duct.

**Seborrhea**-Any increase in scaling of the skin with or without an increase in sebum production.

**Sebum**-The waxy, oily secretory product of sebaceous glands.

**Self**-Molecules and cells that belong specifically to an individual.

**Sporotrichosis**-A fungal infection caused by *Sporothrix schenckii*. which may be transmissible from cats to humans.

**Squamous cell carcinoma**-A malignant, locally invasive, neoplasm derived from either the basal cell layer of the epidermis or the upper epithelial layers of the hair follicle; many but not all squamous cell carcinomas are caused by persistent and prolonged exposure to the sun's ultraviolet light.

**SPF**-Sun protection factor.

**Steroids**-A common name for glucocorticoids. *see* corticosteroids.

**Subcutis (subcutaneous tissue)**-*see* panniculus.

**Systemic Lupus Erythematosus**-An autoimmune disease that causes disease in more than one body organ system.

# T

**Telogen**-Period before hair is shed, resting or final phase of a hair cycle.

**Telogen deflexion (telogen effluvium)**-Hair loss following stressful events such as pregnancy or illness.

**Toxic epidermal necrolysis**-A life-threatening disease involving the mucous membranes and skin., believed by some to be a severe form of erythema multiforme., it is characterized by destruction of skin (necrolysis).

**Transmissible venereal tumor**-A contagious tumor of dogs transmitted by sexual contact and direct contact usually recognized on the penis of male dogs.

**Tricho**-Prefix for hair.

**Trichogram**-Microscopic hair exam.

**Trombiculiasis**-Infestation with chiggers.

**Tumor**-A firm swelling in the skin which may extend into the deeper subcutaneous tissue.

## U-Z

**Ulcer**-A break in the skin's surface exposing the underlying layers of the skin.

**Uria**-Urination, polyuria, increase in urination.

**Uveodermatologic syndrome**-The preferred name for VKH-like disease.

**Vasculitis**-Inflammation of blood vessels.

**Vellus**-Fine hair that follows the lanugo hair.

**Ventrum**-The belly, groin, mammary area, in the case of pets, the underside.

**Vesicle**-An elevation of the epidermis filled with clear fluid.

**Vitamin A-responsive dermatosis**-A skin problem that responds to vitamin A supplementation. Not the same as vitamin A deficiency.

**Vitiligo-**A patchy loss of pigment either hereditary or acquired.

**Vogt-Koyanagi-Harada-like syndrome (VKH)**-An auto-immune disease that affects the pigmented cells of the body.

**Weeping-**Exudation of clear serum form the skin from an inflammation.

**Wheal-**A discreet, raised lesion that disappears within minutes or hours.

**Xanthomatosis**-A papule, nodule or plaque of yellow color in the skin composed of an accumulation of lipids in macrophages/histiocytes known as foam cells.

**Zinc-responsive Dermatosis**-A skin problem that responds to zinc supplementation. Not necessarily the same as zinc deficiency.

**Zoonosis**-A disease communicable from animals to man.

**Zoophilic-**Pertaining to organisms that have adapted to humans, i.e., *Microsporum canis*, one of the causes of ringworm.

# Index

# Suggested Reading

*The following is a list of textbook references which will provide the reader with readily accessible in-depth knowledge, including further reading recommendations.*

*Small Animal Dermatology*, 4th ed., Muller G, Kirk RW, and Scott DW, Philadelphia, W.B. Saunders Co., 1989.

*Veterinary Clinics of North America: Small Animal Practice*, Vol. 20, No. 6, Philadelphia, W.B. Saunders Co., November 1990.

*Veterinary Clinics of North America: Small Animal Practice*, Vol. 18, No. 5, Philadelphia, W.B. Saunders Co., November 1988.

*Veterinary Immunology*, Tizard I, 4th ed. Philadelphia, W.B. Saunders Co., 1992.

*Current Veterinary Therapy-X & XI*, Kirk RW, Philadelphia: W.B. Saunders Co., 1989, 1992.

*Current Veterinary Dermatology*, Griffin CE, Kwochka KW and McDonald JM, Mosby Year Book, 1993.

*Proceedings Second Dermatology World Congress* in Montreal, in press.

*Canine and Feline Endocrinology and Reproduction*, Feldman, E and Nelson, RW. Philadelphia, W.B. Saunders Co., 1987.

*Canine and Feline Dermatology*, Baker & Thomsett, Blackwell, 1990.

*What Every Dog Owner Should Know About Nutrition*, Ackerman, L, Alpine Publications, 1993.

*Tumors of Domestic Animals*, 3rd ed., Moulton, Ed., University of California Press, Los Angeles, 1990.

*Pathology of Domestic Animals*, 4th ed., The Skin and Appendages, Jubb, Kennedy and Palmer, pp. 706-737, Academic Press, Orlando, 1993.

*Veterinary Pathology*, 5th ed., Jones, TC and RD Hunt: The Skin and Its Appendages, pp 1108-1132, Lea and Febiger, Philadelphia, 1983.

*Veterinary Dermatopathology*, Gross T, Ihrke PJ and Walder E, Mosby Year Book, St. Louis, 1992.

*A Beginner's Introduction to Homeopathy*, Cook, TM, Keats Publishing, Inc., 1987.

DermaPet®

## *Registration Information*

**Attention:** Register your book to receive **up to $25 in free credits** to be used toward the purchase of computer discs, supplements (including charts, associated articles and pictures), future books and DermaPet products. Clip this form and send it to DermaPet, PO Box 59713, Potomac, MD 20859.

Name _____

(Business name) _____

Address _____

City_____ State _____ Zip _____

Telephone number (    ) _____

Place of purchase _____